Men's Fitness
magazine

C000112832

7 RULES OF BUILDING MUSCLE

By Joe Warner

Art Editor Richard Davis
Design Ian Jackson, Jo Gurney
Subeditor Juliet Giles
Photography Tom Miles, Duncan Nicholls
Model Kirk Miller@WAthletic

Equipment supplied by escapefitness.com.
Thanks to Fitness First (fitnessfirst.co.uk)

For more information on *Men's Fitness* magazine, go to **www.mensfitness.co.uk**

 © Copyright Dennis Publishing
Ltd. Licensed by Felden 2011 **MAGBOOK**

Publishing Director **Richard Downey**
Managing Director **James Burnay**
Digital Production Manager **Nicky Baker**
Bookazine Manager **Dharmesh Mistry**
Operations Director **Robin Ryan**
Managing Director of Advertising
Julian Lloyd-Evans
Newstrade Director **David Barker**
Chief Operating Officer **Brett Reynolds**
Group Finance Director **Ian Leggett**
Chief Executive Officer **James Tye**
Chairman **Felix Dennis**

The 'MagBook' brand is a trademark of Dennis Publishing Ltd,
30 Cleveland St, London W1T 4JD. Company registered in England.
All material © Dennis Publishing Ltd, licensed by Felden 2011,
and may not be reproduced in whole or in part without the
consent of the publishers.

7 RULES OF BUILDING MUSCLE ISBN 1-906372-70-5

To license this product please contact Hannah Heagney on
+44 (0) 20 7907 6134 or email hannah_heagney@dennis.co.uk

Advertising
Katie Wood katie_wood@dennis.co.uk
Matt Wakefield matt_wakefield@dennis.co.uk

To subscribe to *Men's Fitness* magazine, call **0844 844 0081** or go to **www.mensfitness.co.uk**

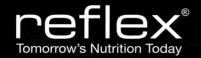

reflex®
Tomorrow's Nutrition Today

+166%

Instant Whey now incorporates Native Whey which is produced by taking fresh skimmed milk and processing it at low temperature via complex ultra and membrane filtration which captures virtually every single highly valuable and biologically active protein fraction in its native form. As a result, it contains up to **166% more bioavailable cystine** which is integral to the production of glutathione, the body's master antioxidant which plays a vital role in immune support and recovery from intense exercise. It also provides up to **16% more leucine** to aid muscle repair and growth.

PERFORMANCE & HEALTH WITHIN

INSTANT WHEY

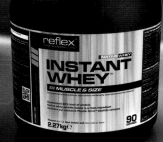

CONTENTS

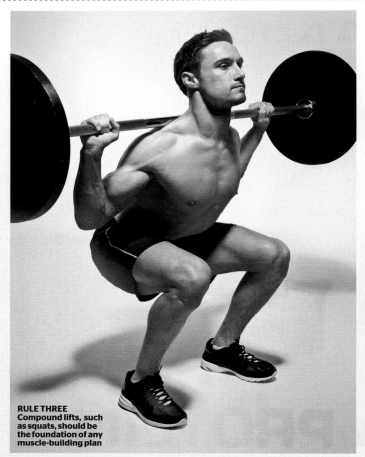

RULE THREE
Compound lifts, such as squats, should be the foundation of any muscle-building plan

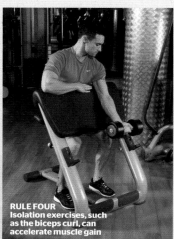

RULE FOUR
Isolation exercises, such as the biceps curl, can accelerate muscle gain

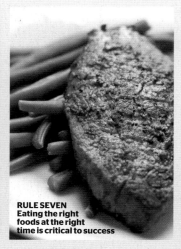

RULE SEVEN
Eating the right foods at the right time is critical to success

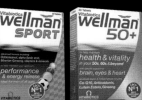

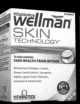
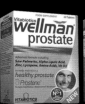

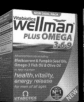
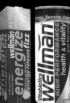

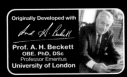

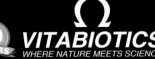

FOREWORD

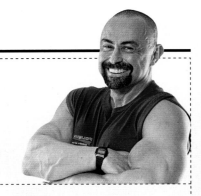

by Charles Poliquin, the world-renowned strength and conditioning coach, who has trained Olympians in 12 sports, world record holders in ten sports and professional athletes in the NBA, NFL, NHL, MLB and English Premier League

>> The chances are that you've picked up *7 Rules Of Building Muscle* for one of several reasons. You may have never set foot in a gym before but want to make some positive changes to your physique. Or maybe you have trained with weights for a while but have been disappointed by your progress. Or you may be an experienced gym-goer who's looking for new ways to continue to add muscular size and strength.

The scenarios may be different, but the ultimate aim is exactly the same. You want to add hard, lean muscle to your frame to be fitter, stronger and to look better with your shirt off. Let's face it – who doesn't?

Despite what you may think, building muscle is easy. That's right. There is no myth or mystery about packing hard, lean muscle to your frame. It doesn't require pills and foul-tasting potions, nor does it involve risking life and limb on all manner of kit and equipment that looks as though it should really belong in a medieval dungeon.

All that's required is that you train smart, eat well and then rest to allow your muscles to build back bigger and stronger. But what type of exercises should you be doing and how often? Why should you shake up your training to ensure your muscles grow? When is the right time to ring these changes? And what are the best foods to fuel muscle performance and recovery?

If you are looking for the answers to these and many more questions about building the body you've always wanted, then you've come to the right place. In your hands you're holding the definitive guide to building muscle, with all the information, tips and advice you need to build your dream body effectively and efficiently.

The only question I have is: what are you waiting for?

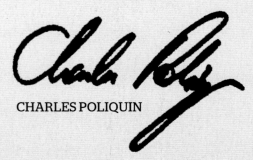

CHARLES POLIQUIN

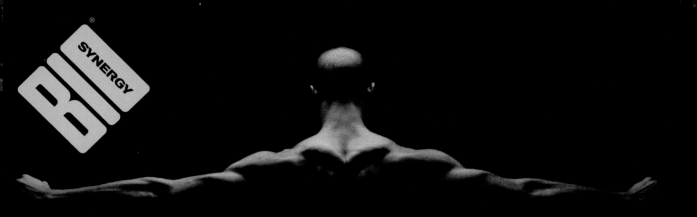
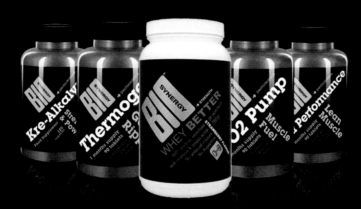

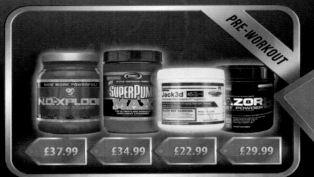
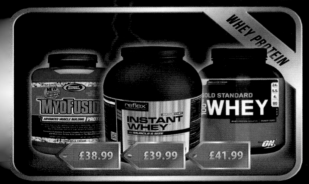
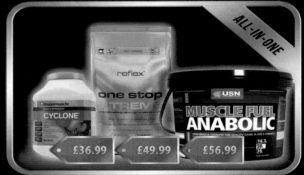
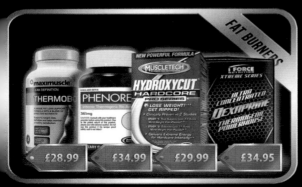
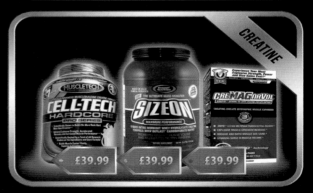

ABOUT THIS BOOK

To build strong, lean muscle faster you need to follow just seven simple rules

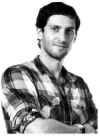

Joe Warner, editor

>> Here at *Men's Fitness* magazine we get asked a lot of questions, and many are on the subject of how best to build muscle. With so much training information flying around – either at the gym, or on websites and online forums – and offering often contradictory ideas on how to make yourself bigger, stronger and leaner, the simple truths can quickly become over-complicated and downright confusing.

Which is why this book has separated the facts from the fiction and the fads to provide you with all the information you need – explained in simple but highly effective terms – on how you can transform your physique into the one you've always wanted.

Simple steps

In the first chapter we help you identify your body type. Once you know this, you can make the most of your strengths – while minimising your weaknesses – to start adding muscle quickly and efficiently. We also detail the muscle groups of the body, explain how they move and the science behind how they grow, and we answer the muscle-building questions we're frequently asked.

In chapter two we give you the tools to assess your current level of fitness and explain why you need to build a strong foundation to make injury-free progress. We then reveal exactly how you can do this, along with a clear guide to warming up, cooling down and stretching – all of which are vital to prevent injury and prime your muscles for growth.

Chapter three focuses on compound exercises – those that involve more than one muscle group – which form the basis of all successful muscle-building training programmes. With our step-by-step guide you'll be able to master these extremely effective moves in no time.

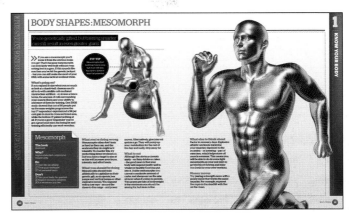

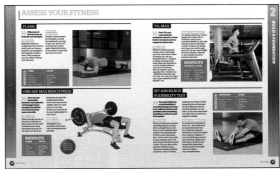

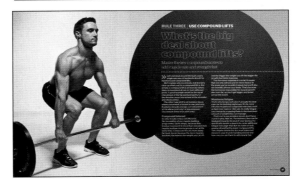

ABOUT THIS BOOK

Mix it up

The next chapter examines the limitations of doing the same exercises week in, week out and details the main variations of the key compound moves and why you should do them to keep your muscles growing. We also look at how you can identify and fix any muscular imbalances or weaknesses that might be holding you back.

Chapter five takes a magnifying glass to the key components of an individual workout – including exercise selection,

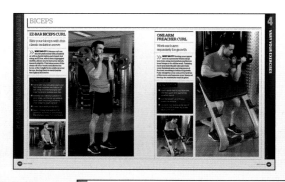

> **'By clearly explaining what you need to do, when to do it and why, we hope to make your muscle-building journey successful and enjoyable'**

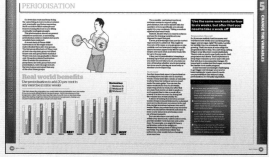

sets, reps and tempo – and why changing these regularly is crucial in the pursuit of bigger muscle.

Chapter six then examines different set strategies and long-term training programmes to help you meet your goals quickly and effectively.

Food for thought

The final chapter is a comprehensive guide to the hugely important role nutrition plays in building and maintaining muscle. We give you the basic rules you need to follow, some easy-to-follow meal plans and handy muscle snacks, along with an in-depth investigation into supplements, such as protein powder, creatine and fat-burners, and tell you if you really need them.

So sit back and start reading. That's the easy bit. Then you can put your newfound knowledge into action. We won't lie: this is the hard part, and it requires motivation, determination and dedication. But by clearly explaining what you need to do, when to do it and why you need to do it, we hope to make your muscle-building journey not only successful, but also enjoyable.

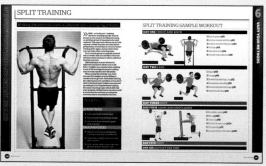

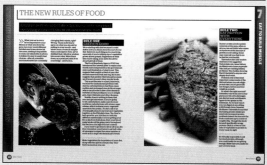

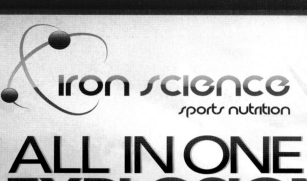

iron science
sports nutrition

ALL IN ONE EXPLOSION

A Cost Effective Yet Great Tasting Protein Powder, without Breaking your Budget

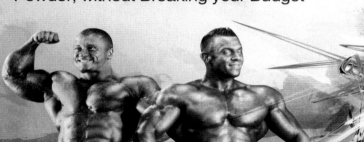

LOWEST PRICE IN THE UK GUARANTEED

» CONSUMERS ONLY
» HIGHEST GRADE

» NO EXPENSIVE PRICE TAGS
» MASSIVE SAVINGS ONLINE

» PRICES CHECKED WEEKLY
» YOU SAVE YOU GAIN

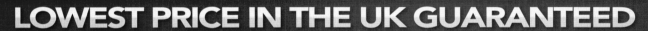

WHEY PROTEIN CONCENTRATE
2.5KG

£25.49
FROM
£7.80 / KG

WHEY PROTEIN ISOLATE
2.5KG

£34.29
FROM
£10.70 / KG

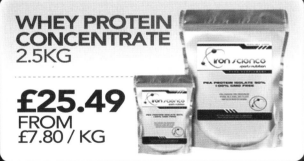

WWW.IRONSCIENCE.CO.UK
BUY DIRECT **0844 544 7992**

FREE DELIVERY
ON ORDERS OVER £35.00

   FANTASTIC VALUE FORMULAS MANUFACTURED UNDER ISO 9001

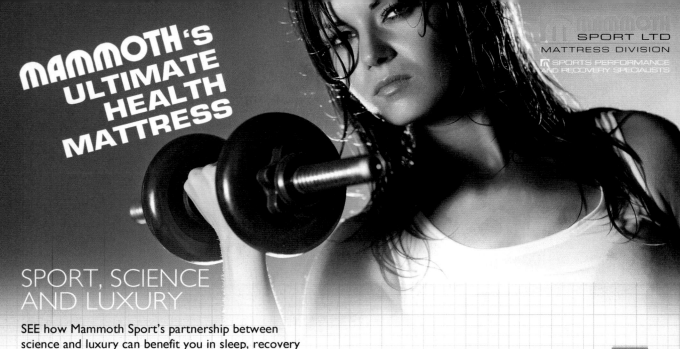
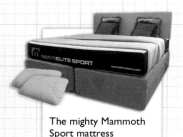
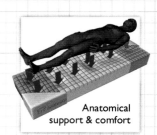
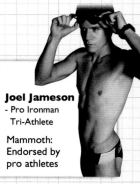
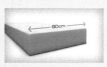
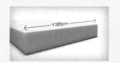
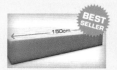
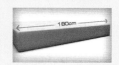
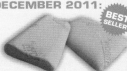
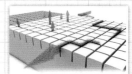

RULE ONE

KNOW YOUR BODY

CONTENTS

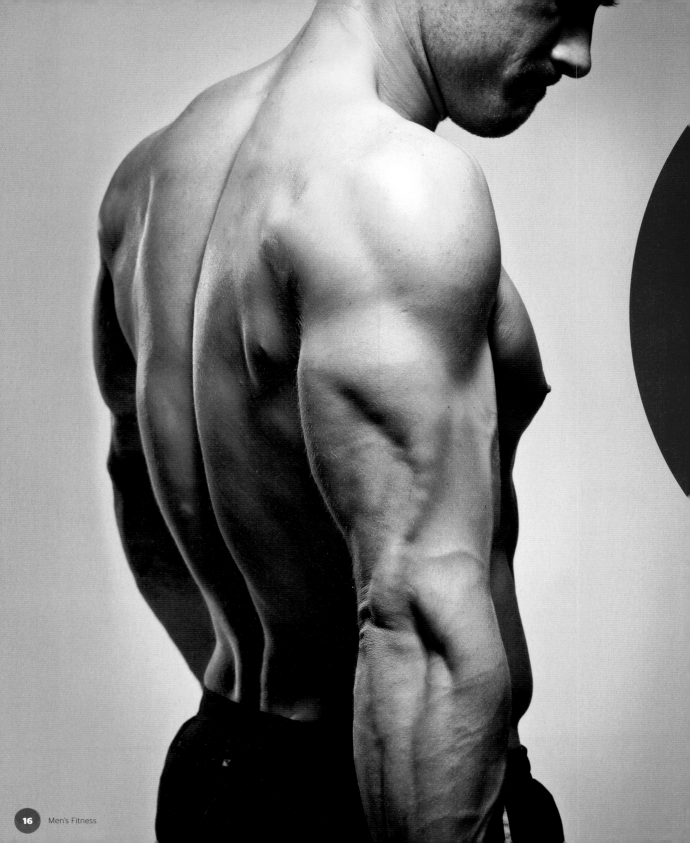

Control your body shape

Whether you pack on muscle easily, struggle to shift your gut or stay lean despite hours lifting weights, smart training will maximise your potential

>> Before we begin it's important that you establish which body shape you have been gifted by your parents. Knowing this means you can train in the most efficient way possible to reap maximum changes in minimum time.

The idea that human body types are genetically pre-set is nothing new. Plato mentions it in *The Republic*, which was written around 380BC, and the 19th-century philosopher Friedrich Nietzsche referred to the idea in *The Antichrist* years before psychologist William Herbert Sheldon popularised three broad 'categories' of body in the 1940s.

But it's since Sheldon's conclusions were published that it has become widely recognised that most people have a body type that marks them out as either being an endomorph (big with high levels of body fat), a mesomorph (muscular) or an ectomorph (lean).

Power struggle

Over the past decade, science has discovered a lot more about how your genetic makeup determines what your body shape will be – and, more importantly, what you can do to overcome your genetic shape. Read on to learn more about the three different body shapes and discover the steps you can take to control your natural shape – rather than let it control you – to get the body you've always wanted, no matter what hand your genes have dealt you.

Are you an endomorph, mesomorph or ectomorph? Turn over to find out.

BODY SHAPES : ENDOMORPH

Shift your spare tyre by ditching cardio for weights and watching what you eat

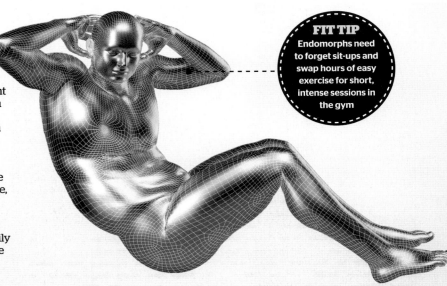

>> If you have trouble shifting weight even when watching your diet, the chances are you're an endomorph, characterised by having a relatively high amount of stored fat, a wide waist and a large bone structure. Great for powerlifters, not so good when you're heading to the beach.

What's going on?

Evolutionarily speaking, you're a badass: when food was scarce, natural selection probably favoured humans with fat-storing metabolisms. But now sofas and milkshakes are readily available, those same genes are scuppering you. In one study where subjects were overfed for 1,000 calories a day over a 100-day period, weight gain varied from 4.3kg to 13kg, and demonstrated that people more predisposed to store fat put on three times as much weight as

FIT TIP
Endomorphs need to forget sit-ups and swap hours of easy exercise for short, intense sessions in the gym

others. Some experts suggest that heredity factors might account for as much as 70 per cent of your body mass index (BMI), so don't be too hard on yourself if the weight isn't coming off. You just need to train smarter.

What you're doing wrong

There's no point in spending hours on a treadmill. If you're trying to lose weight you need to ditch long, slow, steady-state cardiovascular work for more interval-based conditioning to strip away fat. Sprints and box jumps are great, but if you're heavy to the point of being worried about your joints, then moves like the sled push are slower but just as effective. And don't fall into the trap of doing hundreds of sit-ups to shift your gut. The idea you can spot reduce fat is a myth. To reveal that hidden

six-pack you need to lose weight from everywhere.

What you should be doing

You should be combining hypertrophy, or muscle-building work, with conditioning to strip away that unwanted body fat. A four-day split could go something like: Monday, upper-body hypertrophy; Tuesday, lower-body conditioning such as sprints; Thursday lower-body hypertrophy; and a Friday 'repetition' day on the upper body, when you'll do lots of reps at relatively low weights.

What to eat

Unfortunately, you'll have to watch what you eat more strictly than people with other body shapes. The first thing to keep an eye on is the amount of carbs you're eating. Too many

Endomorph

The look
Rotund

Why?
High tendency to store body fat

Do
- ☑ Train with intensity
- ☑ Watch your carb intake
- ☑ Build your shoulders

Don't
- ☒ Do endless sit-ups
- ☒ Jog for hours
- ☒ Drink sports drinks

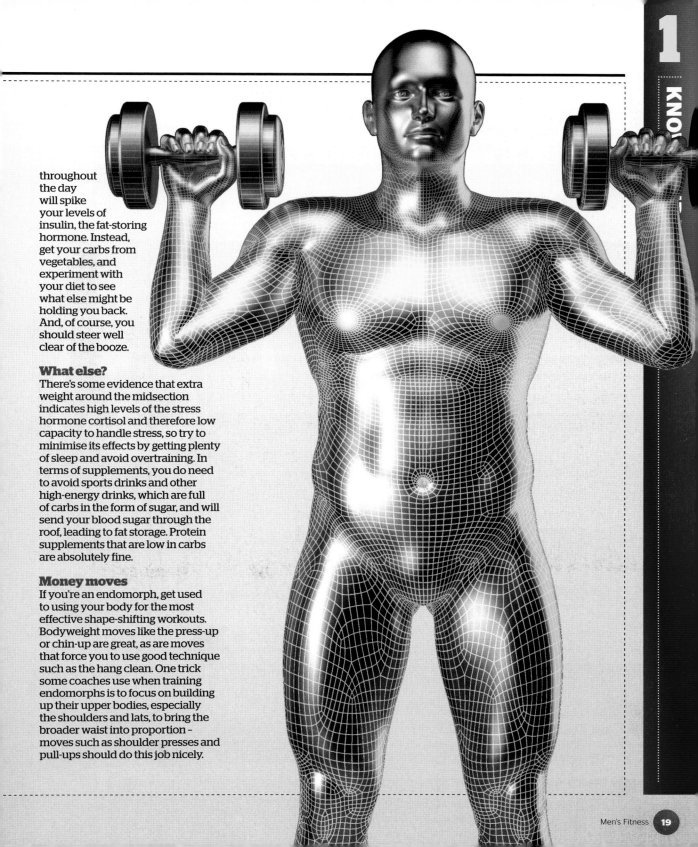

throughout the day will spike your levels of insulin, the fat-storing hormone. Instead, get your carbs from vegetables, and experiment with your diet to see what else might be holding you back. And, of course, you should steer well clear of the booze.

What else?

There's some evidence that extra weight around the midsection indicates high levels of the stress hormone cortisol and therefore low capacity to handle stress, so try to minimise its effects by getting plenty of sleep and avoid overtraining. In terms of supplements, you do need to avoid sports drinks and other high-energy drinks, which are full of carbs in the form of sugar, and will send your blood sugar through the roof, leading to fat storage. Protein supplements that are low in carbs are absolutely fine.

Money moves

If you're an endomorph, get used to using your body for the most effective shape-shifting workouts. Bodyweight moves like the press-up or chin-up are great, as are moves that force you to use good technique such as the hang clean. One trick some coaches use when training endomorphs is to focus on building up their upper bodies, especially the shoulders and lats, to bring the broader waist into proportion – moves such as shoulder presses and pull-ups should do this job nicely.

BODY SHAPES : MESOMORPH

You're genetically gifted, but training smarter can still result in even greater gains

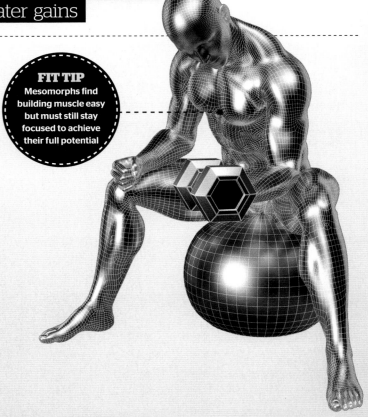

>> If you are a mesomorph you'll know it from the envious looks you get. That's because mesomorphs can look fairly well built without even setting foot in a gym. If this sounds like you then you've hit the genetic jackpot – but you can still make the most of your DNA with some tactical workout tricks.

What's going on?
If you expand in size when you so much as look at a dumb-bell, chances are it's all to do with satellite cell-mediated myonuclear addition – or, in non-science terms, the amount of cells surrounding your muscle fibres and your ability to add more of them by training. One 2008 study showed that out of 66 people put on the same weights programme the top 17 'responders' experienced a 58 per cent gain in muscle cross-sectional area, while the bottom 17 gained nothing at all. If you're a good 'responder' you've got a great head start, but losing fat and training efficiently can work wonders.

FIT TIP
Mesomorphs find building muscle easy but must still stay focused to achieve their full potential

Mesomorph

The look
Well-built

Why?
High metabolism, responsive muscle cells

Do
☑ Train like an athlete
☑ Time your workouts
☑ Set personal bests

Don't
☒ Take your body for granted
☒ Neglect recovery sessions
☒ Eat whatever you like

What you're doing wrong
Mesomorphs often don't train as hard as they can, and the workouts they do might lack intensity. To counter this, try performing timed workouts so that you have a target to aim at as this will increase your focus, intensity and effort levels.

What you should be doing
Mesomorphs should train athletically to capitalise on their genetic gift, so do sprints, box jumps and vertical jumps or other explosive moves. You respond well to low reps – around the three-to-five range – and power moves. Alternatively, give interval sprints a go. They will pump up your metabolism for the rest of the day and really strip away fat.

What to eat
Although the obvious caveats apply – no fizzy drinks or cakes – the good news is that your body will respond pretty well to whatever healthy food you put into it. Unlike endomorphs you can eat a moderate amount of carbs, and always err on the side of more when it comes to protein. Two grams per kilo of bodyweight is the minimum you should be aiming for, but more is fine.

What else to think about

Factor in recovery days. Explosive athletic workouts minimise your muscles' exposure to the eccentric – or lowering – part of exercises, which helps stave off muscle soreness. This means you will be able to do do some light movements on your rest days to get the blood flowing and keep you fresh for your next workout.

Money moves

Try pairing a strength move with a power move that works the same muscles. For example, superset five reps on the deadlift with five on the clean.

BODY SHAPES: ECTOMORPH

It's hard for you to build muscle, but not impossible provided you use big lifts and good carbs

>> You've got the build of a marathon runner – lean, but short on muscle. And it can be difficult to pack on size despite hours in the gym.

What's going on?
Research shows that some individuals have trouble responding to strength training. Further tests on the group mentioned on page 20 showed that the worst 'responders' saw no change in their regulation of myogenin – a key gene responsible for muscle growth – while other subjects on the same workout programme saw their levels spike by as much as 65 per cent. But don't be put off by this. Different people respond better to different training regimes and by tweaking the volume, intensity or frequency of their workouts the poor responders may well have seen better results.

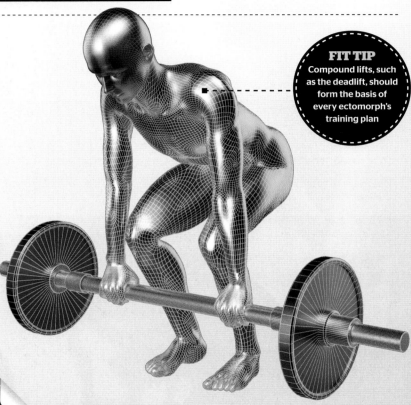

FIT TIP
Compound lifts, such as the deadlift, should form the basis of every ectomorph's training plan

Ectomorph

The look
Lean and long

Why?
Difficulty building muscle.

Do
- ☑ Train with compound moves
- ☑ Eat enough protein
- ☐ Use isolation moves as 'finishers'

Don't
- ☒ Overemphasise isolation moves
- ☒ Train too often
- ☒ Do too much cardio

What you're doing wrong
First, ditch the treadmill: you're lean enough. Long, slow distance work, is the worst thing you can do. Second, don't pack your weights session with classic isolation moves like the biceps curl. You need to build your training programme around big, compound movements like the squat, deadlift and bench press. These involve more muscles and give you the hormonal boost that helps build muscle. You can still use isolation moves, but they need to supplement your main workout: around 80 per cent of your workout should be based on hitting your major muscle groups.

What you should be doing
Compound movements, four sets, in the eight to 12 rep range. But you don't have to live in the gym to put on muscle – quite the contrary. If you're working out four or five days a week then you're making things inefficient because you'll be speeding up your metabolism too much and making it difficult to put on size. Stick to three quality sessions per week and keep the training time, after a warm-up, to 45 minutes or less.

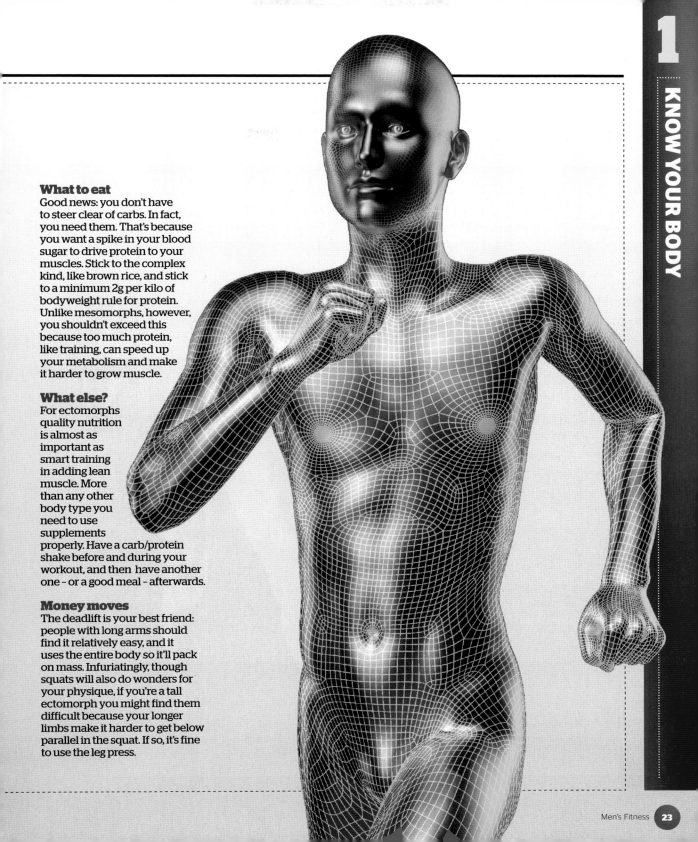

What to eat

Good news: you don't have to steer clear of carbs. In fact, you need them. That's because you want a spike in your blood sugar to drive protein to your muscles. Stick to the complex kind, like brown rice, and stick to a minimum 2g per kilo of bodyweight rule for protein. Unlike mesomorphs, however, you shouldn't exceed this because too much protein, like training, can speed up your metabolism and make it harder to grow muscle.

What else?

For ectomorphs quality nutrition is almost as important as smart training in adding lean muscle. More than any other body type you need to use supplements properly. Have a carb/protein shake before and during your workout, and then have another one – or a good meal – afterwards.

Money moves

The deadlift is your best friend: people with long arms should find it relatively easy, and it uses the entire body so it'll pack on mass. Infuriatingly, though squats will also do wonders for your physique, if you're a tall ectomorph you might find them difficult because your longer limbs make it harder to get below parallel in the squat. If so, it's fine to use the leg press.

KNOW YOUR MUSCLES

There are over 600 muscles in the human body. These are the major ones you'll be targeting during your workouts

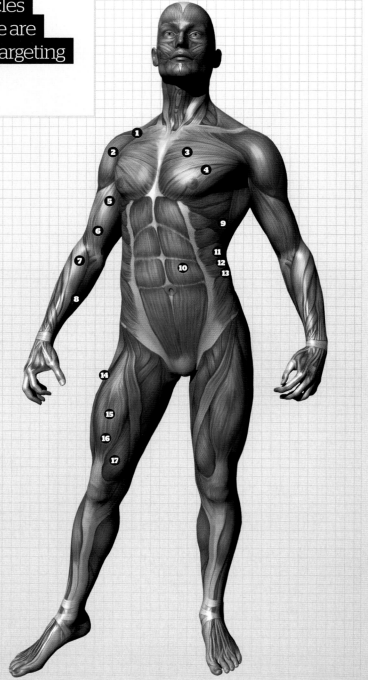

Deltoids
❶ Medial deltoid (middle)
❷ Anterior deltoid (front)

Pectorals
❸ Pectoralis major
❹ Pectoralis minor (beneath the pectoralis major)

Biceps
❺ Biceps brachii
❻ Brachialis
❼ Brachioradialis

Forearms
❽ Flexor carpi radialis

Abdominals
❾ Serratus anterior
❿ Rectus abdominis
⓫ External obliques
⓬ Internal obliques (beneath external obliques)
⓭ Transverse abdominis (beneath internal obliques)

Quadriceps
⓮ Vastus lateralis
⓯ Rectus femoris
⓰ Vastus intermedius (beneath rectus femoris)
⓱ Vastus medialis

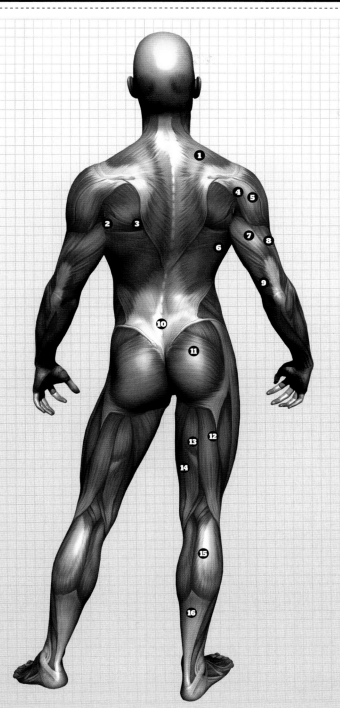

Traps
1 Trapezius

Back
2 Teres major
3 Rhomboid
(beneath
trapezius)

Deltoids
4 Rotator cuff (beneath deltoids)
5 Posterior deltoid (back)

Lats
6 Latissimus dorsi

Triceps
7 Triceps brachii long head
8 Triceps brachii lateral head
9 Triceps brachii medial head

Lower back
10 Erector spinae

Glutes
11 Gluteus maximus

Hamstrings
12 Biceps femoris
13 Semitendinosus
14 Semimembranosus

Calves
15 Gastrocnemius
16 Soleus

MOVE YOUR BODY

How your muscles control every move you make

>> Every time you take a walk, burst into a sprint or lift a barbell off the ground, a huge number of intricately connected and co-ordinated muscle actions take place. It feels so natural that you never even think about it, but every single move you make is changing your body's position on one of several planes and axes. Here's what you need to know.

THE PLANES AND AXIS OF HUMAN MOVEMENT

The three planes

1 Sagittal plane
This passes from front to rear, dividing the body into right and left sections.

2 Frontal plane
Also known as the lateral plane, this passes from left to right at right angles to the sagittal plane, dividing the body into front and back sections.

3 Transverse plane
Also known as the horizontal plane, this divides the body into upper and lower sections.

The three axes

1 Frontal axis
This passes through the body from right to left at right angles to the sagittal plan.

2 Sagittal axis
Also known as the transverse axis, this passes horizontally from front to rear at right angles to the frontal plane.

3 Vertical axis
Also known as the longitudinal axis, this passes from head to feet at right angles to the sagittal plane.

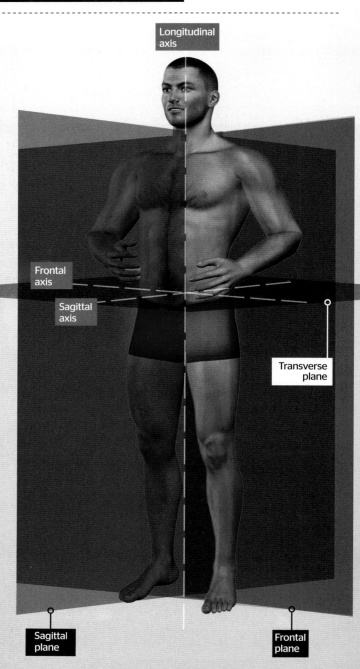

Longitudinal axis

Frontal axis

Sagittal axis

Transverse plane

Sagittal plane

Frontal plane

MUSCLE ACTIONS

All movement begins with a muscle contraction, which pulls on a joint to move your skeleton. These muscle contractions can be categorised into one of three distinct types

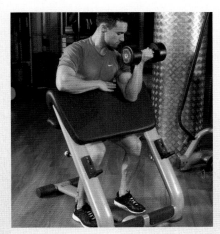

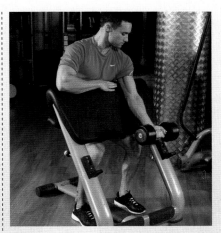

Concentric
During concentric contractions the muscle shortens while generating force. In general, concentric muscle actions are responsible for the 'lifting' part of an exercise, such as the biceps shortening as you lift a dumb-bell to shoulder height during a biceps curl.

Eccentric
During eccentric contractions – usually the 'lowering' part of an exercise – the muscle lengthens and is around ten per cent stronger than it is during concentric contractions. It is these heavy eccentric loads that cause the maximum amount of damage to your muscles. It's for this reason you should always lower a weight slowly and under control: not only does this minimise the risk of injury it also makes each rep more effective.

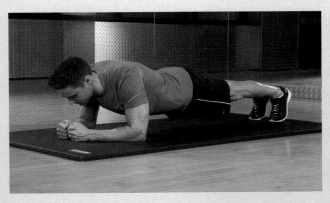

Isometric
During isometric contractions a muscle generates force without changing length. Examples include your entire abdominal region during a plank, or the muscles of the hand and wrist when you grip an object. Although research by NASA into preventing muscle mass breakdown found isometric contractions aren't as effective for building and maintaining muscle mass as concentric and eccentric contractions, they should still form part of your workout, especially for abs and core work. But, isometric contractions can cause a rapid rise in blood pressure so should be avoided if you have a heart condition.

HOW MUSCLES GROW

The simple science behind adding muscle mass

>> Muscle growth is essentially your body responding to the stress of weight training by thinking, 'that was hard, I'd better do something about it so it's not as difficult next time'.

This is because when you perform weight-training exercises you create microscopic tears in your muscles, and your body's response to this 'microtrauma' of the muscle cells is to overcompensate by not just repairing the damaged tissue but adding more. In this way your muscles become bigger and stronger and so the risk of future damage is minimised. It also means you should progressively increase the weight you lift, because your muscles quickly adapt to deal with the stress to which they have been exposed.

It's also thought that this damage to your muscle fibres is the reason for the soreness and stiffness you feel in your muscles in the days after a tough workout, known as delayed onset muscle soreness, or DOMS. And it's why you should leave at least 48 hours between sessions that target the same muscle group. If you train again before your muscles have been repaired and rebuilt you won't be as strong and you run the risk of injuring yourself.

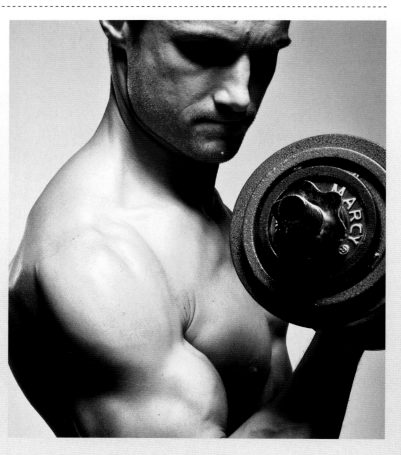

Anatomy of a muscle
Here's what your muscles are made of

>> Muscles are constructed of bundles of fibres contained in protective sheaths, called fascia, which are then bundled together. The biggest bundle is the muscle itself. The next bundles in line are the fascicles, which contain the long, single-celled muscle fibres. Muscle fibres are then sub-divided into myofibrils, which are divided again into bundles of myofilaments, made up from chains of sarcomeres.

1 EPIMYSIUM
A layer of connective tissue that encases the entire muscle.

2 ENDOMYSIUM
A layer of connective tissue that covers the muscle fibres and also contains capillaries (tiny blood vessels) and nerves.

3 PERIMYSIUM
A layer of connective tissue that bundles together

between ten to several hundreds of individual muscle fibres into fascicles.

4 FASCICLE
A bundle of individual muscle fibres.

5 MYOFILAMENTS
The smallest fibre bundles in your muscles.

6 MUSCLE FIBRE
Individual muscle fibres come in two main types:

How muscles work

What happens to your muscles while you workout and rest? These are the key stages in the process of breaking down and rebuilding muscle fibres

1 The warm-up
An increased heart rate pumps blood to your muscles, warming them up and allowing them to extend fully. It also supplies muscle fibres with oxygen.

2 Loading the muscle
At the start of the rep your muscles are under load and stretched. As a result your heart pumps more blood into the protective sheaths that surround the muscle fibres, supplying oxygen and nutrients to these fibres.

3 Sparking your nervous system
When you want to lift the weight your central nervous system relays this fact to the nerves contained in the sheaths protecting the muscle fibres. This in turn tells the muscle fibres to contract, and so lift the weight. If you're doing the exercise correctly, your muscles activate in a particular sequence and your central nervous system adapts to this. As you repeat the workout over time, your nerves get more efficient, so you can do more reps or lift more weight.

4 Chemical reactions
Adenosine triphosphate (ATP) is the immediate energy source for muscle contraction. It is broken down within the body's cells to release energy. The cells' creatine, phosphate and glycogen reserves are also converted into ATP. This process creates lactic acid as a by-product.

5 Feeling the burn
Once glycogen stores in the cells have been depleted and lactic acid has built up, the muscle can't work efficiently, so you need to rest. While you rest, aerobic (oxygen-based) muscle respiration occurs, converting lactic acid back into glycogen to give you energy for the next set.

6 Successful failure
As you reach failure on your last set, your fast-twitch muscle fibres become completely fatigued. Microscopic tears ('microtears') are created in the myofilaments, the smallest fibre bundles in your muscles.

7 Repair and growth
The first way your muscles start to grow is through the post-workout repair process. Your body repairs the microtears by adding the amino acids actin and myosin to the myofilaments, which also causes them to grow in size. The body is unable to grow additional muscle cells, however, so growth is limited by the number of cells that you have. Another effect of intense workouts is that your muscles adapt to store more glycogen, so that there will be more energy on hand for the next workout. This also has the happy side effect of making the muscles increase in size slightly.

type 1 or slow-twitch, which are best suited to endurance because they are slow to fatigue; and type 2 or fast-twitch, which are suited to fast, explosive movements and quickly fatigue.

7 BLOOD VESSEL
Part of the circulatory system, blood vessels come in three types: arteries, which transport oxygenated blood away from the heart; veins, which transport deoxygenated blood and back to the heart; and capillaries, the smallest blood vessels, which enable the exchange of nutrients and waste products between the blood and tissues.

8 TENDON
Strong, connective tissue that connects muscles to bone.

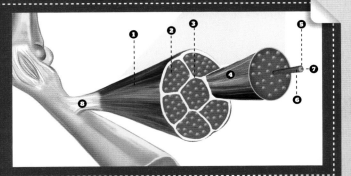

WEIGHT LIFTING GLOSSARY

Here's what those key weight training terms actually mean

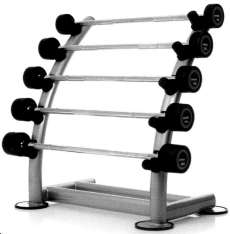

Fixed barbells

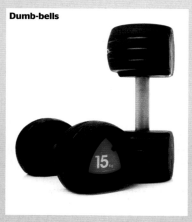

Dumb-bells

Anabolic
A metabolic phase during which nutrients from your diet, specifically protein, are synthesised by your body and turned into muscle tissue.

Atrophy
Muscle atrophy is the wasting away of muscle tissue leading to a decrease in muscle mass, typically due to inactivity.

Catabolic
The opposite to anabolic, this the process by which tissue is broken down and used as energy.

Concentric
The portion of a lift where the muscle shortens under tension – for example, the raising phase of a biceps curl.

DOMS
Delayed Onset Muscle Soreness. This is the dull, ache or pain in a muscle, accompanied by soreness, tenderness and stiffness that is typically felt 24 to 72 hours after strenuous exercise. It is a symptom of muscular damage caused by eccentric movements.

Dumb-bell
One of the best known types of free weight, dumb-bells can be used to add extra resistance to almost every exercise, typically by holding one in each hand.

Eccentric
The portion of a lift where the muscle lengthens under tension – for example, the lowering phase of a biceps curl.

EZ-bar
A type of barbell with a series of kinks in the middle designed to put less pressure on the wrists, forearms and elbows.

EZ-bar

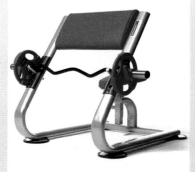

Failure
Performing a set of exercises until you're unable to complete a single extra rep.

Form
The technique used when performing an exercise.

Free weights
Any type of weight training equipment used to increase muscle size and strength. Most common examples include dumb-bells, barbells and kettlebells.

Hypertrophy
Muscle hypertrophy is the growth in the size of your muscle and is

caused when the constituent cells of muscle tissue increase in size as a result of a stimulus, such as weight training.

Intensity
The intensity of any set you perform is determined by the weight you're lifting and expressed as a percentage of your one-rep max.

Kettlebell
Originating from Russia, these cast-iron balls of different weights have a handle on top so you can grip them with one or two hands while performing different exercises.

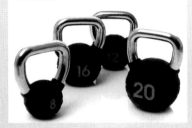

Kettlebells

Range of motion
The full extent or range of a muscle's movement. Performing lifts through your muscles' full range of motion is important in muscle growth.

One-rep max
The maximum amount of weight you can lift once with correct form. A good method for measuring your absolute strength.

Olympic barbell
The Olympic barbell is used for all manner of lifts. They have thick 'sleeves' for the weights to slot on to, which means they can spin when you're doing lifts such as the clean

or snatch. A full-length bar weighs 20kg. Fixed barbells don't spin, so they're better for moves using lighter weight.

Overtraining
When over exertion leads to injury, muscle strain or fatigue.

Rep
One complete movement of a given exercise. Abbreviation of repetition.

Resistance machines
These allow you to target specific muscles in a pre-determined path of movement. Favoured by novices and bodybuilders, machines reduce the risk of injury because of their set range of motion, but they don't work your small, vital stabilising muscles.

Rest
The period of recovery time in between sets and exercises.

Set
A number of reps performed consecutively without rest. Can vary from one rep to more than 20, depending entirely on training goals.

Smith machine
A weight-training frame comprising a barbell that slides up and down on a fixed plane of motion. You lower the barbell on to a series of hooks on the frame to stop it moving, meaning you can lift heavy weights without a squatter. Normally used for squats and bench presses.

Squat rack
A frame used to hold a weighted barbell. Unlike a Smith machine, the

barbell isn't connected to the frame so you can move it through more than one plane of motion and have to use more muscles to keep it stable.

Spotter
Someone who assists you with a lift, especially towards the end of a set, to ensure you can complete each rep safely.

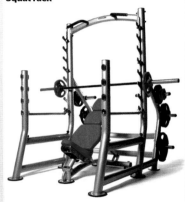

Squat rack

Supercompensation
Period of adaptation following a tough workout when your body recovers and gets stronger. Correctly timed training, recovery then training again will result in increases in muscle size and strength.

Superset
Two exercises performed back-to-back with no rest in between.

Volume
Volume is the amount of sets and reps you do for an exercise, a muscle group, or a workout. Increasing training volume is (generally) good for hypertrophy, but it's also a common cause of overtraining.

MUSCLE Q&A

No-nonsense answers to the fundamental fitness questions

Q I've failed to add muscle in the past. Why will it work now?

A If your efforts have been unsuccessful in the past it has nothing to do with your body being fundamentally resistant to exercise and everything to do with your approach. In other words, you haven't had a focused plan so you've not set realistic, achievable goals, and you haven't been eating the right foods. Anyone can make positive changes to the way they look, but not overnight. Going to the gym once or twice a week won't give you a radical transformation, especially if you don't work hard or aren't eating well.

Q Can I turn my body fat into muscle?

A Fat and muscle are two totally different types of tissue so it's impossible for one to turn into the other. Muscle is active tissue that burns calories, while fat tissue stores excess energy. When you train hard you burn away fat and build muscle, giving an appearance that one has turned into the other, but this is not the case.

Q How often do I need to work out?

A Less frequently than you might think. And it's certainly not the case that more is better. That's because it's when you're recovering that increases to your muscle size and strength take place. If you don't take recover sufficiently you won't see improvements. It's not just your muscles that need time to recover; your nervous system is working hard to recruit your muscles, something it's not used to doing, so it also needs time to recover.

Q How long should each workout last?

A The perfect workout should take less than an hour to complete, including warm-up, warm-down and stretching. Research suggests that levels of the growth hormone testosterone peak around 45 minutes into a workout and then quickly subside as levels of cortisol, the stress hormone that breaks down muscle tissue and damages cells, rise. So keep workouts short and effective.

Q Do crunches build a six-pack?

A You can perform hundreds of crunches every day and have the strongest abs in the world but if they're under a layer of fat then you're not going to see them. And if you're trying to burn fat, crunches are just about the worst move you could choose. In fact, you'd have to do about 500,000 of them to burn 1kg of fat. That's about four weeks of solid crunching.

Q Are machines better than free weights?

A Resistance machines have their place in a gym: they're a great way for beginners to learn movement patterns without the risk of injury, and they allow experienced trainers to isolate specific muscles to lift more weight. But because the movement pattern is restricted, they won't work the stabilising muscles that are so important in staying injury free. Using free weights may require more skill, but it will recruit those stabilising muscles and better prepare your body for other activities, especially sports.

Q How quickly will I see results?

A Even with the help of this book, don't expect overnight success. You need to lift heavy weights regularly to stimulate the muscle into growing, eat a clean diet full of high-quality protein and carbs and get plenty of sleep. It's a big commitment.

Q Aren't squats bad for my knees?

A Performed incorrectly, any move is dangerous, but squats have a particularly bad reputation. But a correct squat – in which your feet are shoulder-width apart, and your knees stay in line with your toes – places emphasis on the quads, glutes and hamstrings, and not on any joints. This can reduce the risk of injury by strengthening the muscles and supporting tissues around the knee joint.

Q Are lighter weights best for toning?

A 'Toning' is one of the most popular words in the exercise world. It is also one of the most redundant. You can't 'tone' a muscle, only build it or maintain it, while stripping away fat to give it a more prominent appearance. So when people say they want to 'tone up' they actually mean that they want to add muscle, lose fat, or a bit of both.

FIT TIP
It's best to have a check up with a GP before you begin training.

Q How effective are bodyweight moves?

A If you're new to resistance training, or returning from injury, bodyweight moves are the perfect preparation for heavier lifts. They can also be used effectively as part of supersets or bodyweight circuits, and are far better at building strength and stability in your joints and core than resistance machines.

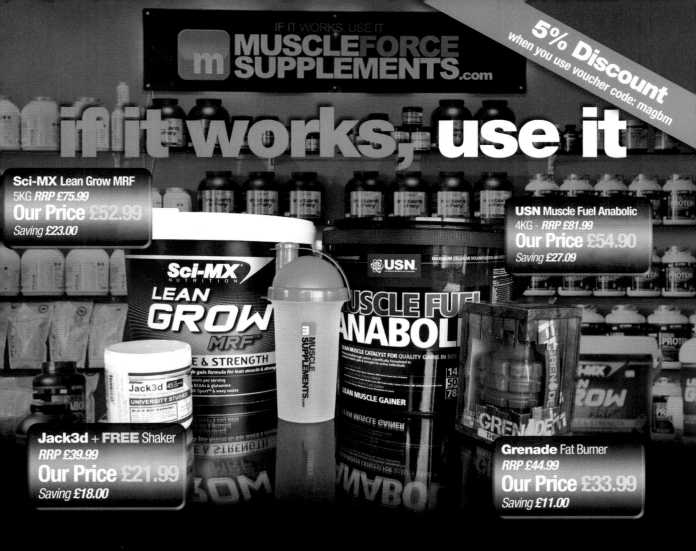
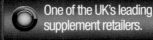
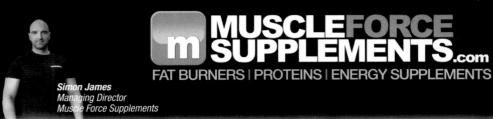

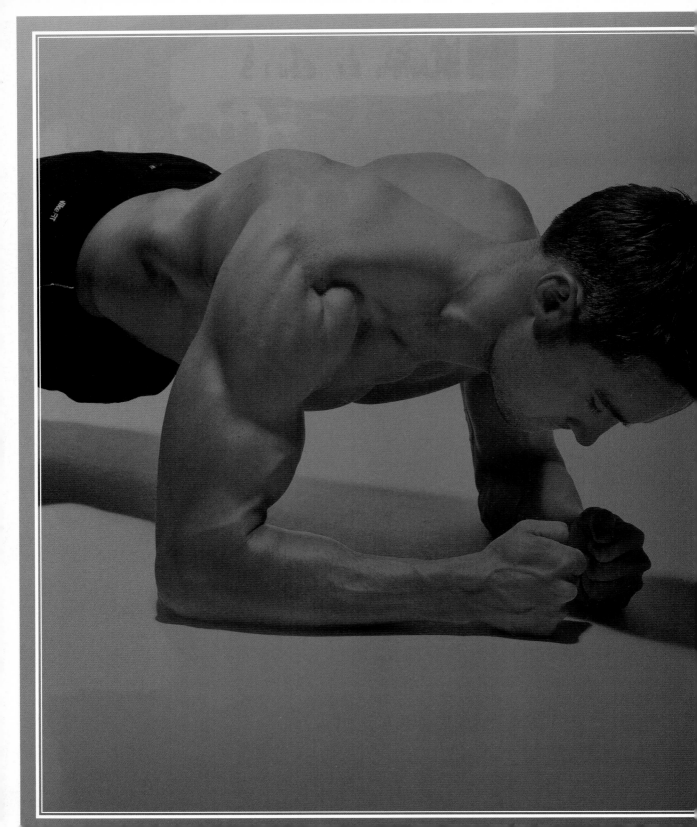

RULE TWO
BUILD A FOUNDATION

CONTENTS

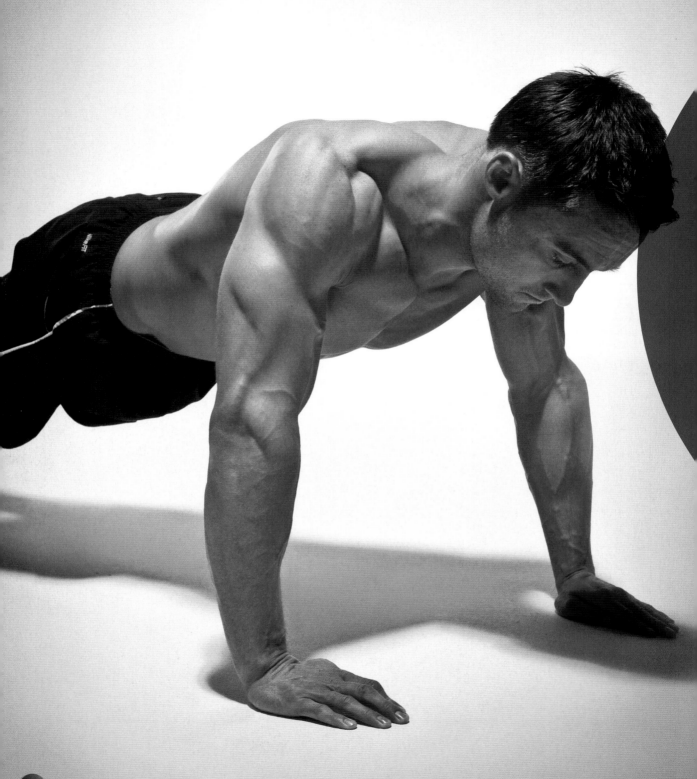

Why do you need a strong foundation?

Create a solid base to make adding muscle easy

>> Building muscle is like building a house. Lay the right foundations and you can build a strong, stable structure that will withstand whatever is thrown at it. But if construction begins without a solid base then you'll end up with a weak, unbalanced frame that is at risk of falling apart.

The good news is that getting a solid foundation for your muscle-building mission is easy.

This chapter explains how, through performing bodyweight exercises (those that rely on your own weight as resistance, such as press-ups), core exercises (which target your abdominal muscles, including your six-pack), and proper warming-up, cooling-down and stretching, you can lay some solid foundations that will make putting on hard, lean muscle far easier.

Why? Because bodyweight moves target the small, but vitally important stabilising muscles that make your joints stable, mobile and healthy, while a strong core supports your torso and assists the transfer of power from your legs to upper body – crucial for the successful completion of almost all standing exercises – especially the shoulder press, deadlift and squat – without injury. The more stable your body, the heavier you'll be able to lift and the faster you'll pack on muscle. So if you want a body that's more Taj Mahal than Leaning Tower of Pisa, read on.

To master the most important bodyweight moves, turn over.

BODYWEIGHT MOVES

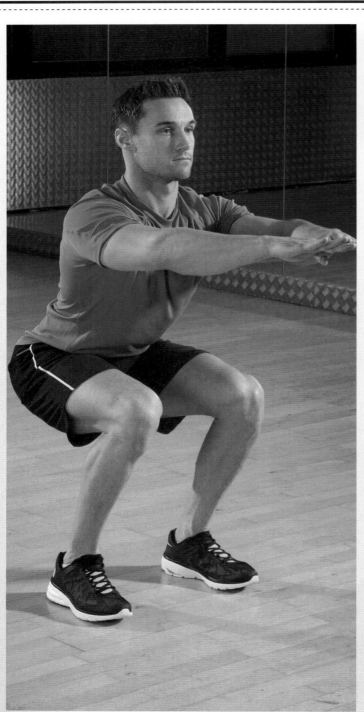

Master bodyweight moves to build muscle, prevent injury and generate explosive power

>> If your aim is to pack on muscular size and strength, it can be tempting to head straight for the weights and start doing bench presses and squats rather than press-ups, lunges and other bodyweight exercises. And that's because most people assume that they are too easy to be effective in building muscle.

But bodyweight moves are great for building a strong and stable foundation of muscle and the fact that you can do them anywhere and at any time is just one of their many benefits. These moves can reduce your risk of injury, they're a perfect way to warm up and they'll improve your ability to go heavier when you do finally hit the weights.

FIGHTING FIT

Take press-ups. They're great at targeting the small muscles of the delicate shoulder joint. Strengthen these stabilising muscles and you'll be able to push heavier and harder on the bench press.

But don't just take our word for it. Many athletes in combat sports make bodyweight moves a key compoment of their training programmes.

Any form of training done by boxers and MMA fighters to prime their muscles for explosive speed and strength is good enough for us. For these athletes, getting a ripped body is just a bonus.

PRESS-UP

>> **The ultimate upper-body test, press-ups require your chest, shoulders and triceps to work hard to lower, then lift, your torso from the floor.**

TARGET
▌Chest
▌Shoulders
▌Triceps

HOW TO DO IT

● Start with your hands shoulder-width apart and body straight.

● Lower yourself until your elbows reach 90°, then press back up.

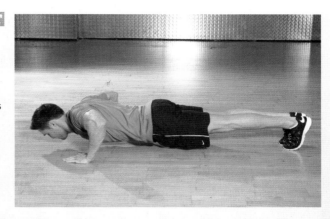

T PRESS-UP

>> **This twist on the classic move requires upper-body co-ordination and a strong core to rotate upwards.**

TARGET
▌Chest
▌Shoulders
▌Triceps
▌Core

HOW TO DO IT

● Start in press-up position and lower chest to ground.

● Press up powerfully and at the top of the move lift one arm off the ground while twisting your torso until that arm points to ceiling.

● Lower back down before repeating on the other side.

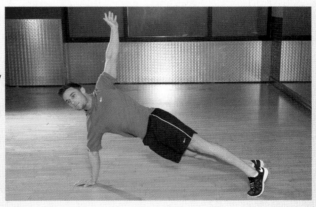

CLAP PRESS-UP

>> **Having to clap in between press-ups means you have to push up from the floor quickly, turning it into an explosive muscle-building move.**

TARGET
▌Chest
▌Triceps
▌Shoulders

HOW TO DO IT

● Start in press-up position and lower chest to ground, keeping elbows close to your side.

● Press back up powerfully so that your hands leave the floor. Quickly clap them together.

● Land back down and descend into the next rep.

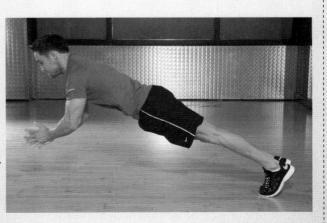

BODYWEIGHT MOVES

SQUAT

>> Mastering the correct form of a squat means you'll make quicker progress when adding additional weight using a barbell or dumb-bells.

TARGET

- Quads
- Hams
- Glutes

HOW TO DO IT
- Stand tall with feet shoulder-width apart and toes pointing slightly outwards.
- Keeping your core braced and a natural arch in your back, squat down until your thighs are parallel to the floor before pushing back up through your heels.

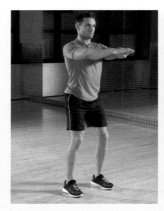
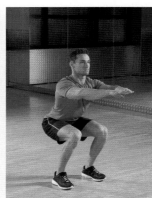

JUMP SQUAT

>> Jumping turns the squat into a powerful plyometric move that fires up your fast-twitch muscles fibres and gets your heart pumping.

TARGET

- Quads
- Hams
- Glutes
- Calves

HOW TO DO IT
- Stand tall with feet shoulder-width apart.
- Squat down, then push back up powerfully so your feet leave the floor.
- As you land descend straight back into a squat and repeat.

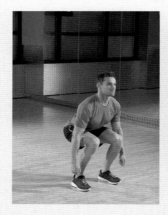
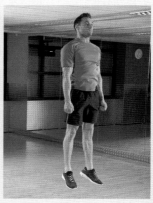

BENCH DIPS

>> Build mass on the back of your arms with this surprisingly tough move.

TARGET

- Triceps
- Shoulders

HOW TO DO IT
- Grip the edge of a bench with your back and legs straight.
- Slowly lower your body straight down, keeping your elbows pointing back throughout, before pressing back up powerfully.

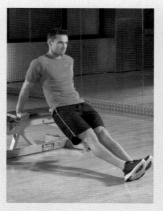
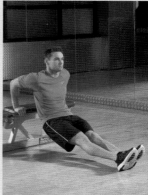

LUNGE

>> Another classic move that requires power, balance and co-ordination.

TARGET

❚ Quads
❚ Hamstrings
❚ Glutes

HOW TO DO IT

● Stand tall with feet apart, chin up, core braced and natural arch in your back.

● Take a step forward and lower your body by bending both knees to 90°. Ensure your front knee doesn't go past your foot.

● Push back off your front foot to move back to the start.

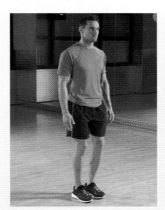
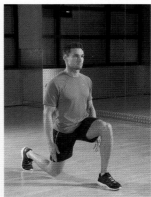

LATERAL LUNGE

>> The often-ignored muscles of your inner thighs are vital for turning movements, both in the gym and on the sports pitch.

TARGET

❚ Adductors (inner thighs)

HOW TO DO IT

● Stand with feet close together, with core braced.

● Take a big step to one side, keeping a natural arch in your back and torso upright. Bend the other knee to lower your body, keeping that knee in line with your foot.

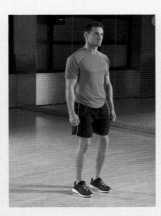
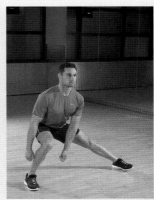

INVERTED SHOULDER PRESS

>> The best way to work your shoulders without weights, this move also requires a strong core and good co-ordination.

TARGET

❚ Shoulders
❚ Triceps

HOW TO DO IT

● Start with your feet on a bench and hands shoulder-width apart on floor, so your body forms an inverted V-shape.

● Slowly lower your body until your face almost touches the floor before pushing back up powerfully.

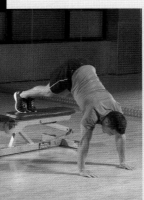
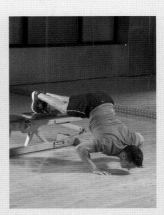

CORE STRENGTH

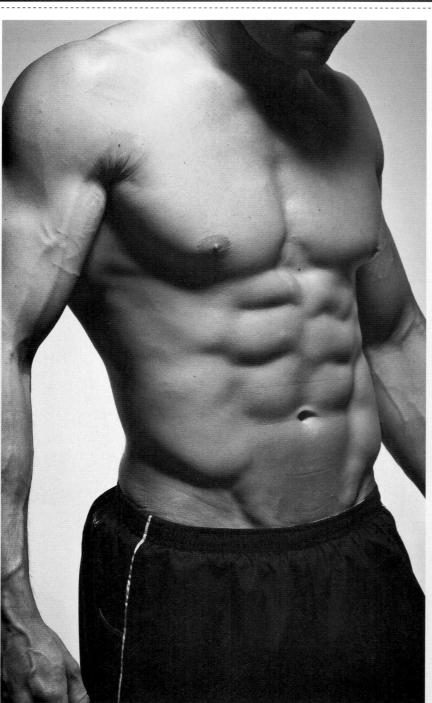

Build a solid midsection and reap the rewards

>> A solid core is more than just about having an impressive six-pack. In fact, having a stomach of steel offers far more benefits to your muscle-building ambitions than just looking good. That's because a strong, stable core means you can more effectively transfer power between your upper and lower body – vital for lifting heavy weights – as well as providing a solid base for almost every upper-body lift, especially those that involve lifting a weight overhead, such as the shoulder press or overhead squat.

Here are eight kit-free moves that target your abdominals, obliques and all the other important deep-lying muscles that make up your core.

CRUNCH

>> **The classic move for targeting your upper abs – and still one of the best.**

TARGET

| Upper abs

HOW TO DO IT

- Lie on a mat with your knees bent at 90° and your feet flat on floor. Place your fingers by your temples.

- Contract your abs to curl your chest towards your knees, keeping your lower back on mat. Squeeze your abs at the top then return to the start.

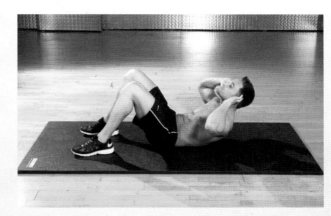

REVERSE CRUNCH

>> **Place the emphasis on the lower part of your abs by hitting them from a different angle.**

TARGET

| Lower abs

HOW TO DO IT

- Lie with your arms by your sides with knees bent at 90° and feet flat.

- Contract your abs to lift your hips off the mat, then curl your knees towards your chest, keeping your knees at 90°. Pause then slowly lower your legs back to the start.

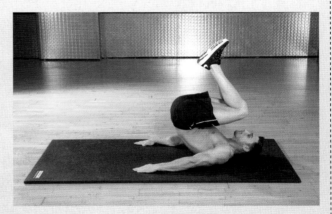

OBLIQUE CRUNCH

>> **Hit your abs from the side to target your obliques – the muscles that frame your six-pack.**

TARGET

| Obliques

HOW TO DO IT

- Lie on your side with one arm in front of body and the other bent so your fingers touch your temples.

- Crunch up sideways and hold for a second at the top of the move and then lower slowly back to the start.

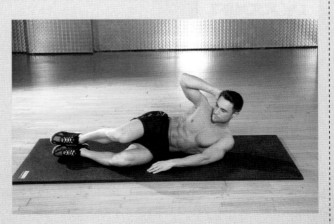

CORE STRENGTH

PLANK

>> **Build a strong link between your upper and lower body.**

TARGET

▌Core

HOW TO DO IT

- Hold your body in a straight line from head to heels with your elbows beneath your shoulders, feet together and face looking down.
- Hold the position for as long as you can without letting your hips sag.

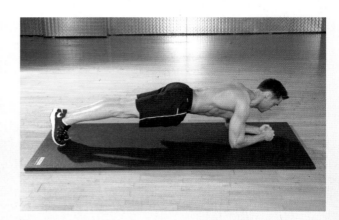

SIDE PLANK

>> **Hold your body straight to build a powerful core and improve your posture.**

TARGET

▌Core
▌Obliques

HOW TO DO IT

- With your elbow directly beneath your shoulder, hold your body in a straight line from head to feet.
- Hold the position for as long as you can without letting your hips sag, then repeat on the other side.

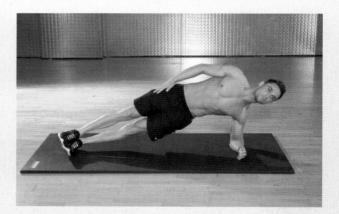

JACKKNIFE

>> **An advanced move that requires flexibility as well as a strong core.**

TARGET

▌Abs

HOW TO DO IT

- Lie flat on your back with your arms behind your head, and your feet together.
- Contract your abs so your hands and feet meet over your stomach. Keep your legs straight and squeeze you abs at top of move then return to the start.

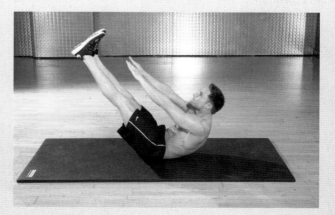

LOWER-BODY RUSSIAN TWIST

>> Keep the focus on your lower abs and obliques with this advanced move.

TARGET

▮ Lower abs
▮ Obliques

HOW TO DO IT

● Lie flat on your back with your arms out to the sides and your legs straight up in the air. Keep your shoulders and upper back on the mat throughout.

● Twist over to one side, keeping your legs straight. Go as far as you can to the side without letting your feet hit the floor. Reverse back to the start and twist the other way.

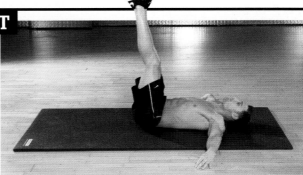

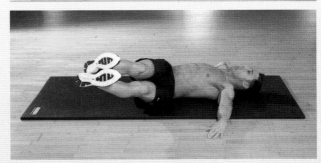

BICYCLES

>> Do them quickly – but in a controlled manner – to really work your core muscles hard.

TARGET

▮ Abs
▮ Obliques

HOW TO DO IT

● Lie flat on your back. Crunch up and bring your right elbow to meet your left knee. Repeat on alternate sides.

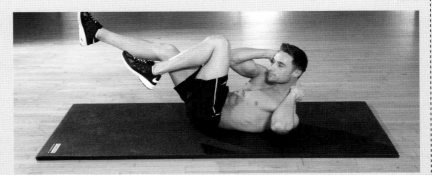

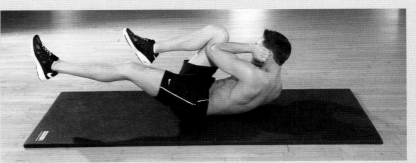

PRE-WORKOUT WARM-UP

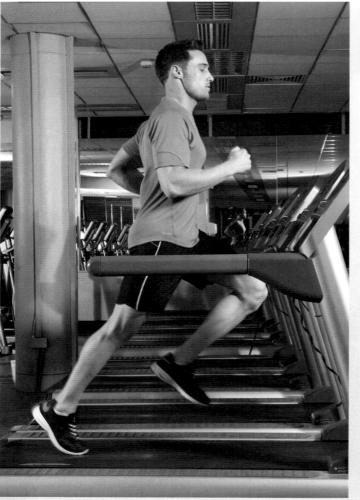

Warm up before every workout to prepare your body and prevent injury

>> A proper warm-up is vital before doing any weight training. If time is short, don't be tempted to skip the warm-up and go straight to your workout, because cold muscles can get easily damaged. A few minutes spent on a warm-up can prevent days lost while recovering from injury.

Your warm-up should start with some light cardiovascular exercise, such as running, rowing or cycling. This will make your heart beat faster, pumping oxygen and nutrients to your muscles, and elevate your body's core temperature. Warm muscles are more elastic than cold ones, so you can work them through a wider range of motion with fewer injuries.

After the cardio you then need to target your muscles directly with dynamic stretches. These differ from static stretches (see next page) in that you are moving as you stretch out the muscle. The trick is to start very gently and then slowly increase the range of motion you use with each repetition. This prepares your muscles and joints for the work to come.

Finally, before you begin any lifting exercise, perform the movements with minimal weight to teach your muscles how to respond when you do the exercise with heavier weights.

WARMING UP

>> Whatever method of cardio you choose, keep the pace gentle and constant. By the end of ten minutes you should be sweating and puffing a bit, but not out of breath.

Cardio 10 minutes >>

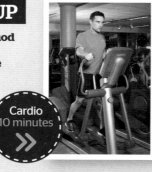

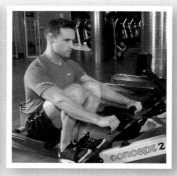

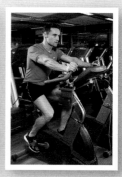

DYNAMIC STRETCHES

After your cardio warm-up perform 10 reps of each of these moves

LUNGE WITH REVERSE FLYE

- Step forward while stretching your arms to the sides.
- Keep your body upright.
- Lunge lower with each rep.

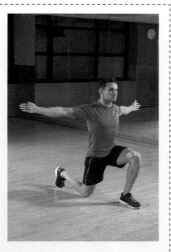

LATERAL LUNGE WITH TWIST

- Step to the side with both feet pointing forward.
- Twist your torso in the direction of your leading foot.
- Bend your knee a bit further with each rep.

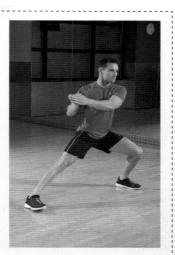

ALTERNATING SPLIT DEADLIFT

- Step forward with one foot and lean forwards from the hips.
- Keep your back straight.
- Lower your hands down your shins a bit further each time, before pushing back to the start.
- Repeat with other leg.

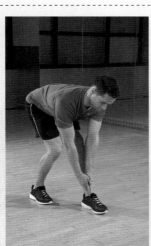

SQUAT TO OVERHEAD REACH

- Stand with feet shoulder-width apart and back straight.
- Squat down and then reach overhead as you stand up.
- Squat a bit lower with each rep.

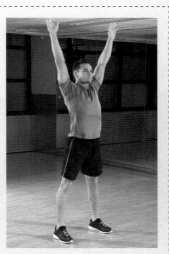

COOLING DOWN

It's important after your final set to cool down before beginning your post-workout stretches (see next page). Cooling down is the process of gradually reducing your heart rate from its elevated state during the main part of your session and also slowly bringing down your core body temperature. Spend five to ten minutes performing some very gentle cardio, gradually reducing the intensity every minute to transition your body back to its resting state.

POST-WORKOUT STRETCHES

Stretch your muscles after each session to improve flexibility

>> With a static stretch you hold a relaxed muscle under tension. This helps lengthen the muscle, which will have contracted after weight training, and provides several benefits. First, it will help with flexibility, so you'll be able to work your muscles across a wider range of motion, leading to bigger muscle gains. But stretching also helps reduce injuries as your muscles and tendons are less likely to tear when they are relaxed.

Stretching also improves blood flow to your muscles, helping to flush out toxins, meaning you'll be ready for your next workout sooner. And stretching can also aid posture, because tense muscles can pull your spine, shoulders and hips out of alignment, leading to a stooped look and lower back pain.

Your muscles need to be fully warmed up before you perform static stretches, so never do them at the start of a workout. To avoid injury, don't pull too hard when you stretch, and don't 'bounce' the muscle under tension.

Hold each stretch for 20 to 30 seconds

STATIC STRETCHES

CALVES
● Push down on your rear heel.

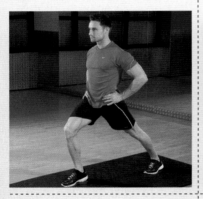

HAMSTRINGS
● Lean forward at the hips with a straight back.

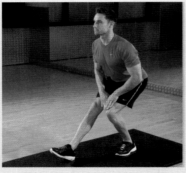

QUADS
● Pull on your ankle and push your hips forward.

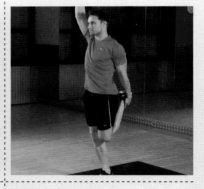

HIP FLEXORS
● Keep your body upright and push your hips forward.

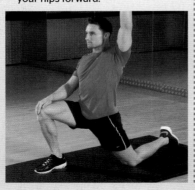

ADDUCTORS
● Press your knees apart gently with your elbows.

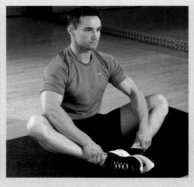

GLUTES
● Gently pull on your knee.

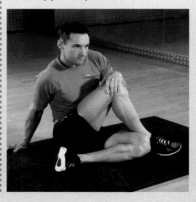

ABS

- Lift your shoulders high off the floor.

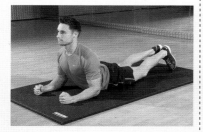

LATS

- Press your shoulder towards the floor.

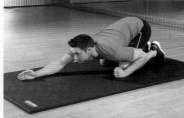

LOWER BACK

- Keep your shoulders flat on the floor.

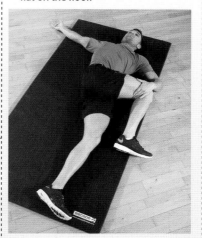

CHEST

- Interlock your fingers and raise your hands behind you with straight arms.

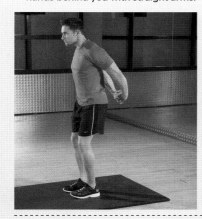

UPPER BACK

- Interlock your fingers and raise your hands in front with straight arms.

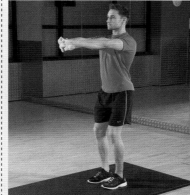

TRAPS

- Pull gently on your head.

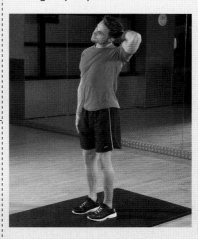

TRICEPS

- Point fingers of one arm down your back and pull gently on that elbow.

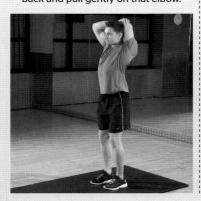

BICEPS

- Press your arms back while twisting your hands so your thumbs point behind you.

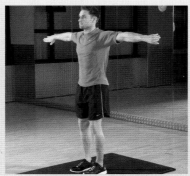

ASSESS YOUR FITNESS

Now you know the main bodyweight moves and how to warm up and warm down, it's time to test your current fitness and strength levels. Turn over to begin.

ASSESS YOUR FITNESS

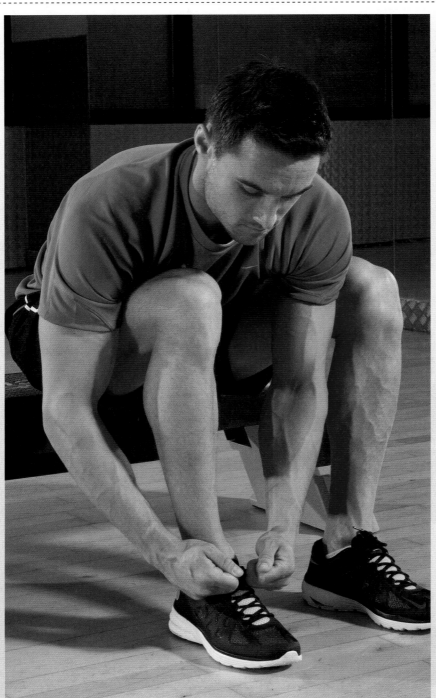

Take these tests, then use our tips to improve your scores

>> Doing these six tests is useful for two reasons. First, they will give you a good idea of your current level of fitness, and they show you in which areas you are weaker and need to improve. That's why each test has some simple 'how to improve' tips included. Second, they will give you a set of concrete numbers against which you can measure your progress. So when you revisit these tests in a month or two you'll see exactly how much fitter and stronger you have become.

PRESS-UPS

» **The humble press-up is an excellent test of upper-body strength and endurance.**

THE TEST

Perform as many press-ups as you can, following the correct form set out on p39. The test ends as soon as you can no longer complete a rep with correct form.

HOW TO IMPROVE

Aim to do three or four sets of max reps, with around 60 seconds' rest between sets. You can also vary the tempo: come down slowly and explode up, for example, and work up to clap press-ups or even slapping your chest as your hands come off the floor to build explosive power.

RESULTS	
SCORE	**LEVEL**
40+	Excellent
30-40	Very good
20-30	Good
10-20	Average
Below 10	Poor

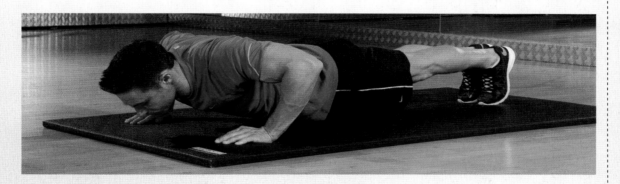

ONE-REP MAX SQUAT

» **The maximum weight you can lift for one rep is the key indicator of lower body strength. See p58 for how to perform the squat correctly.**

THE TEST

Warm up. Ideally, do the test in a squat rack, not on a Smith machine. Aim for four attempts, with three to five minutes' rest in between, increasing the weight between 2.5kg and 10kg each time. Your score is the heaviest weight you can lift with perfect form divided by your bodyweight.

HOW TO IMPROVE

You need to learn to sit back into the squat, keep the weight distributed over your heels and don't let your knees drift too far forwards. It's also worth working on your weak points – lower back, glutes and hamstrings. Try good mornings or Romanian deadlifts.

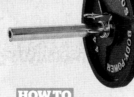

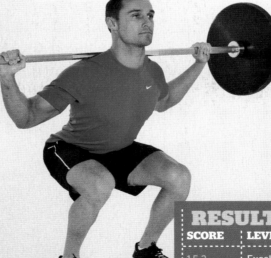

RESULTS	
SCORE	**LEVEL**
1.5-2	Excellent
1.25-1.49	Very good
1-1.24	Good
0.75-0.99	Average
Under 0.75	Poor

ASSESS YOUR FITNESS

PLANK

>> **This is one of the best ways to evaluate core strength.**

THE TEST

Keep your body in a straight line from head to heels with your elbows beneath your shoulders, feet together and face down. Hold as long as you can without letting your hips sag.

HOW TO IMPROVE

Practice makes perfect for the plank, so hold the position for as long as you can. Rest for 30 seconds, then hold it again. Repeat this three or four times a week and see your time soar.

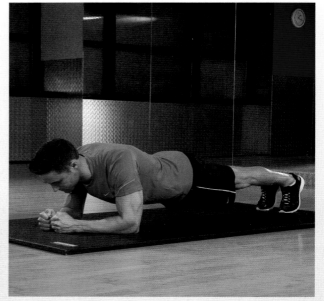

RESULTS	TIME	LEVEL
	2min+	Excellent
	90-119sec	Very good
	60-89sec	Good
	40-59sec	Average
	Less than 40sec	Poor

ONE-REP MAX BENCH PRESS

>> **Your one-rep max on the bench is a key indicator of total upper-body strength. See p60 for how to perform the move correctly.**

THE TEST

With an empty bar, lie on the bench with feet on floor. Lower the bar until it touches your chest then press back up. Do ten reps as a warm-up.

Gradually increase the weight, performing one or two reps at each weight, until you reach your one-rep max. Divide your heaviest lift by your bodyweight for your score.

HOW TO IMPROVE

Strengthen your shoulders and triceps with overhead presses and dips.

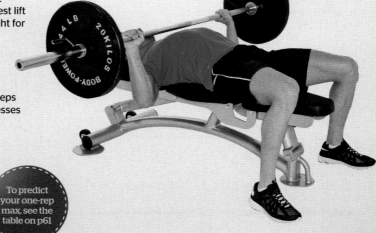

To predict your one-rep max, see the table on p61

RESULTS

SCORE	LEVEL
1.50+	Excellent
1.25-1.49	Very good
1-1.24	Good
0.75-.099	Average
Under 0.75	Poor

VO₂ MAX

>> **Your VO₂ max represents the maximum capacity of your body to transport and use oxygen in a given time.**

THE TEST

Without sophisticated kit, a basic way of estimating your VO_2 max is the Cooper 12-minute run. Set up a treadmill with a 1° gradient to mimic running on the road. Warm up, then aim to run the farthest distance you can in 12 minutes. After 12 minutes, use the equation VO_2 = (metres run - 505)/45 to calculate your VO_2 max. So, if you ran 2.4km your score would be (2,400-505)/45 = 42.

HOW TO IMPROVE

Try doing continuous aerobic training at a heart rate of 70-85 per cent of your maximum (MHR) for 30 to 60 minutes, three to five times a week. To take your fitness up a level, you need to get up to 80-90 per cent of MHR for three minutes, with one or two minutes recovery between intervals.

RESULTS

VO₂ MAX	LEVEL
70 or over	Excellent
60-69	Very good
50-59	Good
40-49	Average
Under 40	Poor

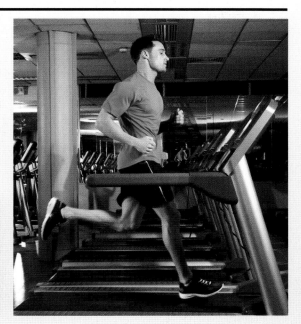

SIT AND REACH FLEXIBILITY TEST

>> **It's a good indicator of the flexibility of your hamstrings and lower back, without which you'll probably pull a hamstring sprinting or end up in pain from squats.**

THE TEST

Warm up with some dynamic stretching before you start. Mark a straight line on the floor as your baseline. Mark another line perpendicular to this as your measuring line – this is where your ruler or tape measure goes. The point where the two intersect is 0cm. Put your feet on the baseline, 20-30cm apart. Clasp your thumbs together and slowly reach forwards, keeping your fingers on the measuring line as you lean forward. Measure how far past the baseline you can reach. If you can't reach past your feet, then you'll have a negative reading.

HOW TO IMPROVE

It's extremely important to warm up – any cardio that increases the heart rate – for at least ten minutes beforehand and then stretch your muscles. However, if you're stretching as part of your workout, always do it afterwards. Research has shown that doing static stretches before strength work can reduce your strength levels.

RESULTS

DISTANCE	LEVEL
15cm or more	Excellent
10-14cm	Very good
0-9cm	Good
-5-0cm	Average
Less than -5cm	Poor

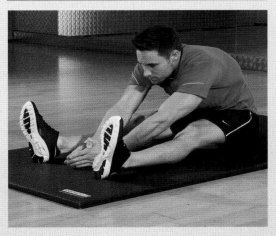

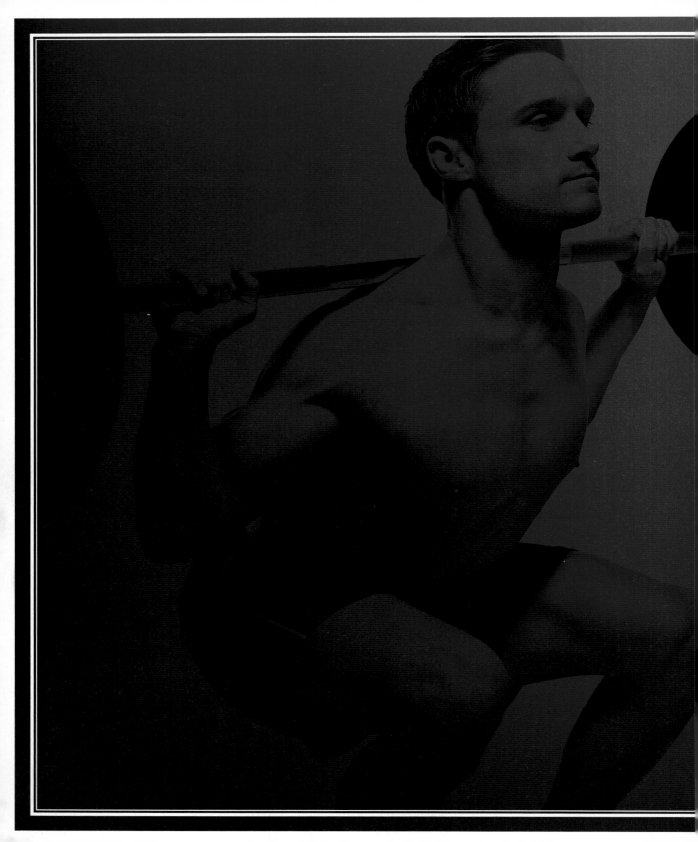

USE COMPOUND LIFTS

CONTENTS

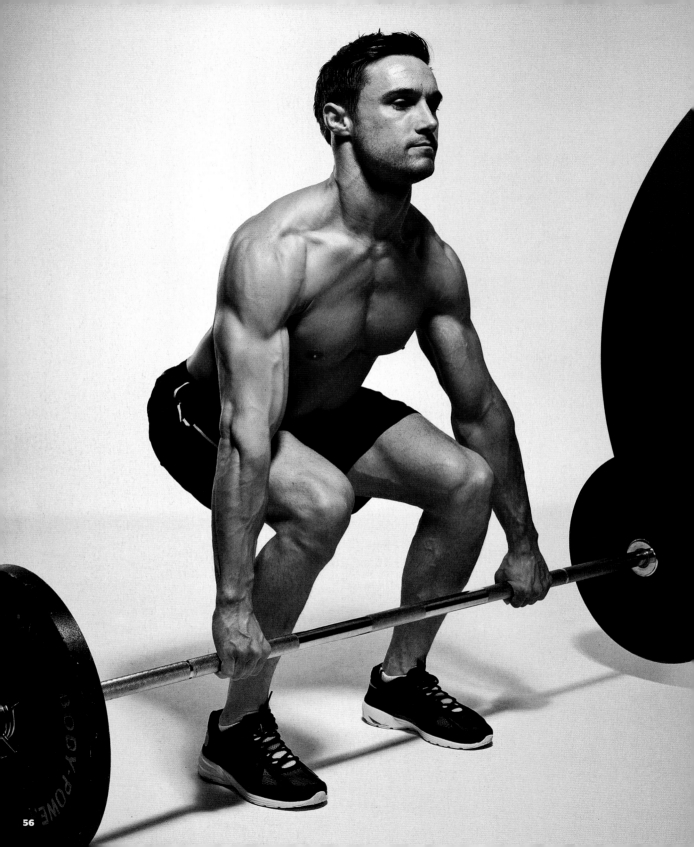

What's the big deal about compound lifts?

Master the key compound moves to add muscle size and strength fast

» Let's not beat around the bush: every single one your of workouts should be based around compound lifts.

We'll explain why in a minute, but first let's clear up what exactly a compound lift is. Put simply, a compound lift is an exercise where there is movement at two or more different joints. A good example would be the squat (movement at the hip and knee joints) or the shoulder press (movement at the shoulder and elbow joints).

The other type of lift is an isolation move, where movement is limited to one joint only. Examples include a biceps curl (movement at the elbow joint only) or leg extension (movement at the knee joint only).

Compound interest

So why should compound lifts form the foundation of any muscle-building programme? Quite simply, because they involve movement at more than one joint they require multiple muscle groups to act at the same time. Compound lifts are more-bang-for-buck moves because the more muscles involved, the heavier the weight you can lift, and the bigger the weight you lift the bigger the growth-hormone response.

This hormone response is crucial. It means that not only will you put on more muscle in the areas you've recently trained, but you'll also see benefits all over your body. That's because the hormones responsible for muscle growth also burn fat, so you'll get bigger *and* leaner across the board.

Maximum fatigue

That's why biceps curls aren't actually the best exercise for building big biceps. It's far more effective to perform compound exercises, such as bent-over rows or chin-ups, to really fatigue your biceps by exposing them to the maximum amount of weight they can manage.

That's not to say isolation moves don't have a part to play, they do. For instance, they can be deployed towards the end of your workout to specifically isolate a muscle to cause additional fatigue (see page 102). But the basis of each session should be the major compound lifts. This chapter details the ten most important moves in your muscle-building arsenal and how you can use them to add muscle fast.

SQUAT

Master this classic move to pack on muscle not just on your legs, but also on your upper body

>> The king of the lifts, the squat targets the quads, glutes, hamstrings, core and back, making it one of the most important exercises – if not *the* most important – in your muscle-building arsenal. Although your legs are the obvious target, squats create an overall anabolic environment that triggers the release of extra testosterone and growth hormone in the bloodstream. This not only benefits your leg muscles but will also help build your upper body and burn fat.

Target

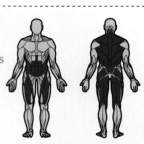

▌Quads
▌Hamstrings
▌Glutes
▌Core
▌Back

How to do it

● Rest the bar against the back of your shoulders – not on your neck – and hold the bar with an overhand grip wider than shoulder width.

● Your feet should be shoulder-width apart with your toes pointing slightly outwards.

● Slowly lower yourself down – keeping your chest and chin up while maintaining a natural arch in your back. Keep the weight on your heels, your body upright and don't let your knees roll inwards or forwards.

● Bring your body down until your thighs are at least parallel to the floor. The deeper you can squat, the better.

● Drive back up through your heels. At the top push forward with your hips and squeeze your glutes to 'reset' into the start position and repeat.

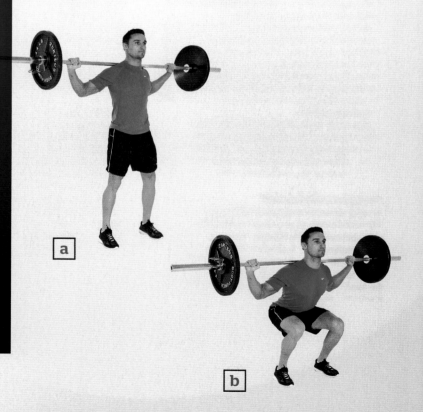

a

b

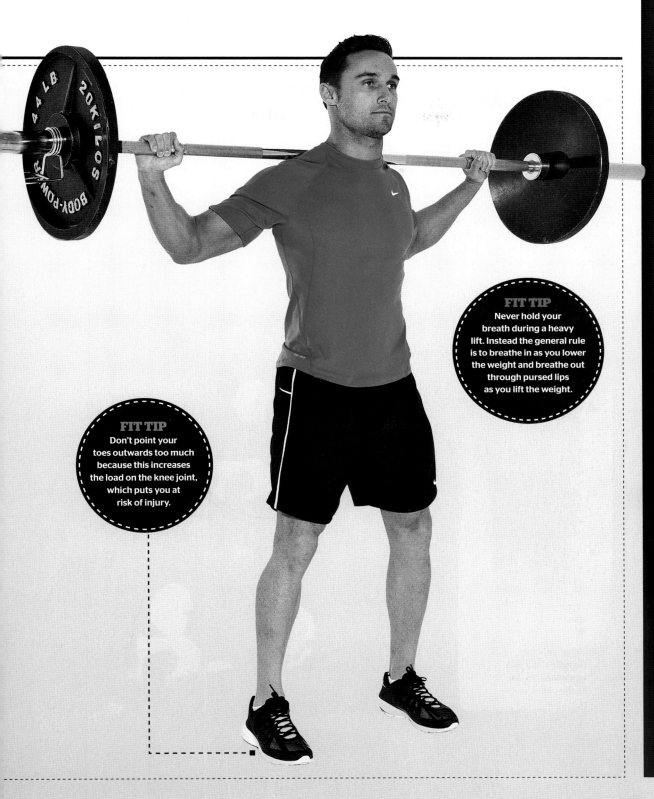

FIT TIP
Never hold your breath during a heavy lift. Instead the general rule is to breathe in as you lower the weight and breathe out through pursed lips as you lift the weight.

FIT TIP
Don't point your toes outwards too much because this increases the load on the knee joint, which puts you at risk of injury.

BENCH PRESS

This big lift will add muscular size and strength the your chest, shoulders and arms

>> The bench press has always been an important and popular move because it is the best exercise for developing upper-body muscular size, power and strength. Mainly working the pectoral, or chest, muscles, this exercises also recruits the muscles at the front of the shoulders and back of the arms, making it a firm favourite for those wanting a big, strong torso. Always warm up thoroughly first with some press-ups then some bench presses with an empty bar.

Target

- Chest
- Shoulders
- Triceps

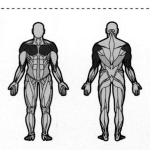

How to do it

- Lie on the bench with your feet on the floor, directly beneath your knees.

- Your head, upper back and glutes should be flat against the bench. Brace your core and maintain a natural arch in your back.

- Hold the bar with an overhand grip that is wider than shoulder-width apart.

- Slowly lower the bar to your chest, taking your elbows out to 90°, until the bar is almost touching the middle of your chest or just over your nipples.

- Drive your feet hard into the floor and press the bar back to the start position.

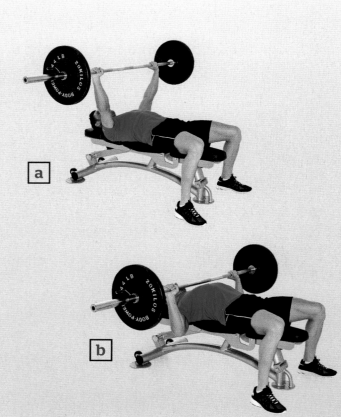

a

b

FIT TIP
A too-narrow grip on the bar places greater emphasis on the triceps (back of your arms). A wider grip shifts more focus on to your chest, but this position makes it harder to achieve a full range of motion.

FIT TIP
Maintain control of the weight throughout the move to keep the focus on your muscles. Bouncing the bar off your chest is not only dangerous but means you're relying on momentum, not muscle.

PREDICTING YOUR ONE-REP MAX

If you haven't got a spotter, don't want to risk a max lift, or have no idea what your max should be, you can use the table below to predict it. Just use a weight that you can do two to ten reps with for a max set, then multiply it by the value on the right to get your predicted max.

EXAMPLE If you can lift 85kg for 5 reps, your predicted 1RM is 85 x 1.18 = 100kg

COEFFICIENT TABLE

REPS	COEFFICIENT
2	1.07
3	1.12
4	1.15
5	1.18
6	1.21
7	1.24
8	1.27
9	1.30
10	1.33

DEADLIFT

This important move allows you to lift heavy and grow serious muscle – so long as you do it right. Here's how

>> The deadlift works wonders on your physique because so many important muscle groups are involved in the move, specifically the legs, glutes and back. Performed correctly, this lift is one of the best exercises for developing a strong and supportive lower back, and because so many muscles are recruited you'll be able to lift a lot of weight. As well as the mass-building benefits of the deadlift, a strong lower back and core will be better at stabilising your upper body during every other move you do, so you'll be able to lift heavier during other exercises too.

Target

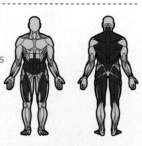

- Quads
- Hamstrings
- Glutes
- Back
- Core

How to do it

- Squat down and grip the bar just outside your knees with your core braced, your shoulders retracted and over the bar and your back flat.

- Use your legs to power the initial lift, pushing down through your heels.

- Keep the bar close to your body and, as it passes your knees, push your hips forward. Keep your shoulders back throughout the move.

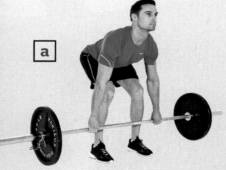

a

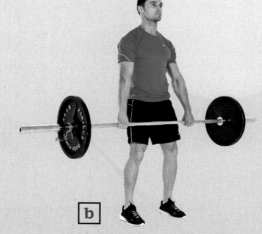

b

+ GET A GRIP

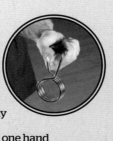

Do you find that your grip is failing before your legs and back to cut every deadlift set short? Poor wrist strength can result in poor performance in many big lifts, so try the barbell collar grip. Hold a collar in one hand and squeeze it for two seconds before releasing slowly. Do this ten to 12 times before swapping hands.

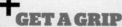

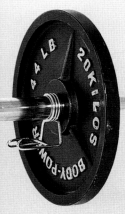
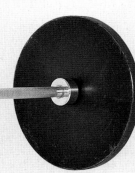

FIT TIP
Keep your core muscles braced throughout every single rep to keep your upper-body stable and prevent lower-back pain.

FIT TIP
Start with a light bar and master the correct deadlift form before gradually adding more weight as you become stronger.

PULL-UP

Raise your game with this upper-body muscle sculptor

>> It may technically be a bodyweight exercise, but the pull-up is one of the hardest moves there is. That's because you have to lift and control your entire body weight against gravity, so the load on your muscles is very high. This has the huge advantage of building a strong, wide upper back, which helps create the V-shape torso women love. Preventing your legs from swinging during this exercise also means that your core muscles get a good workout.

Target

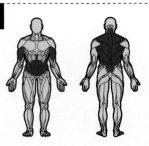

- Back
- Lats
- Biceps
- Core

How to do it

- Grasp the bar using an overhand grip with your hands wider than shoulder-width apart. The wider they are, the harder the move becomes.

- Start from a dead hang with your arms fully extended.

- Pull yourself up by squeezing your lats together.

- Once your chin is higher than your hands, slowly lower yourself back to the start position.

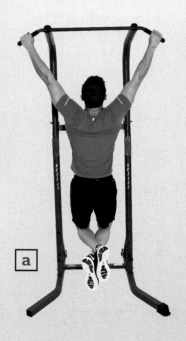

a

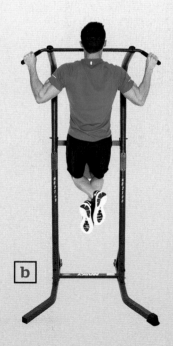

b

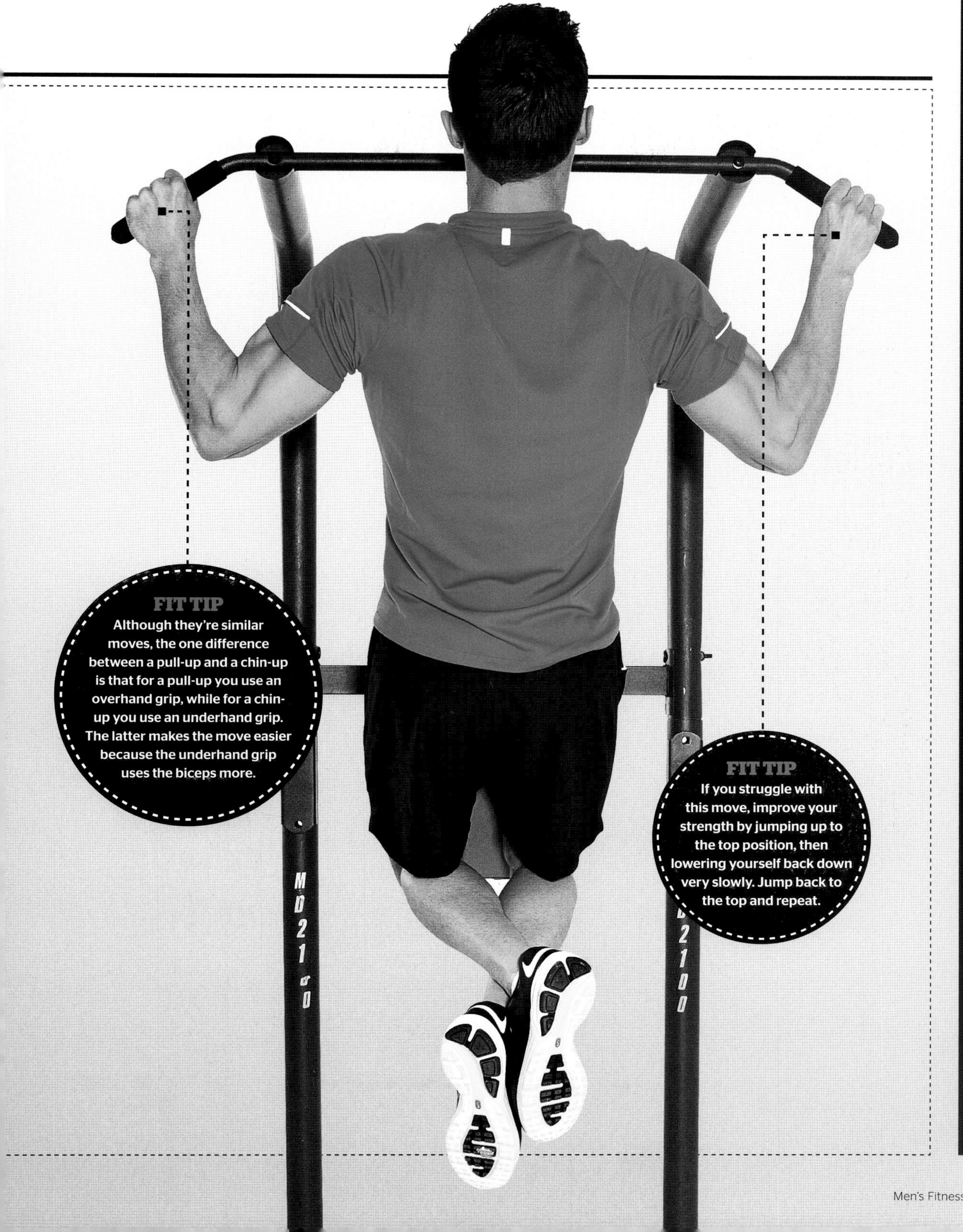

FIT TIP

Although they're similar moves, the one difference between a pull-up and a chin-up is that for a pull-up you use an overhand grip, while for a chin-up you use an underhand grip. The latter makes the move easier because the underhand grip uses the biceps more.

FIT TIP

If you struggle with this move, improve your strength by jumping up to the top position, then lowering yourself back down very slowly. Jump back to the top and repeat.

LUNGE

Build strong, powerful legs and a rock hard core with this tried and tested muscle builder

>> When building strong legs most people overlook lunges in favour of squats, but lunging is one of the most basic human movement patterns. Lunges work the powerhouse lower-body muscles, such as the glutes, quads, hamstrings and calves, but also involve the adductors, hip flexors and many other stabilising muscles – including your core – that need to be strong if you're going to move with speed, power and co-ordination. So not only are they great for building muscle, they also have huge transferable benefit to almost every sport.

Target

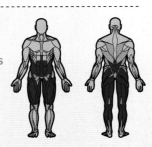

- Glutes
- Hamstrings
- Quads
- Calves
- Core

How to do it

- Stand tall with a barbell resting on the back of your shoulders. Point your elbows behind you to retract your shoulder blades and keep your back upright and core braced throughout.

- Take a big step forward but keep your knee over your front foot and not beyond it. Lower down until both knees are bent at 90° before pushing back off your front foot to return to the start position.

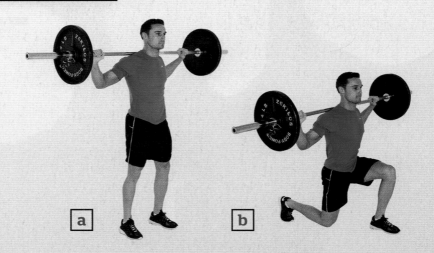

a

b

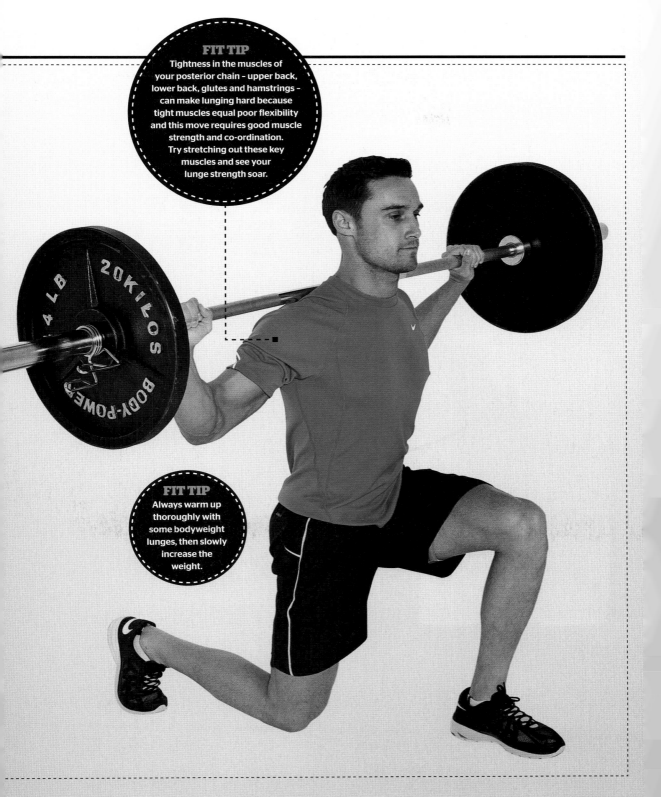

FIT TIP
Tightness in the muscles of your posterior chain – upper back, lower back, glutes and hamstrings – can make lunging hard because tight muscles equal poor flexibility and this move requires good muscle strength and co-ordination. Try stretching out these key muscles and see your lunge strength soar.

FIT TIP
Always warm up thoroughly with some bodyweight lunges, then slowly increase the weight.

SHOULDER PRESS

Develop strong and wide shoulders with this bulk-building upper-body move

>> The shoulder press is a massively important lift for adding size and strength to your upper body. It mainly works the front and middle deltoids – two of the three major muscles that make up your shoulders – but also recruits those small, but very important, stabilising muscles that support the shoulder joint. Your triceps become involved as you straighten your arms, while your core must work hard throughout to stabilise your torso. It's a key move for creating wide shoulders and will help improve your bench press.

Target

I Shoulders
I Triceps

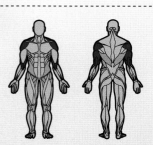

How to do it

- With your feet shoulder-width apart, position a bar on your upper chest, gripping it with hands just wider than shoulder-width apart.

- Keep your chest upright and your core muscles braced.

- Press the bar directly upwards until your arms are fully extended overhead.

- During the lifting phase, keep your core braced and don't tilt your hips forward.

- Lower the bar back down to your chest and repeat.

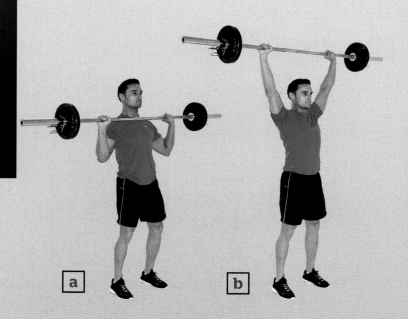

a

b

FIT TIP
The shoulder is one of the most complex joints in the body and not one you want to injure. Always thoroughly warm up the muscles before attempting any heavy lifts.

FIT TIP
The first rep will be the toughest because there's no bounce effect from the elasticity of the muscles, but don't be put off. Use your legs to help initiate the first rep and the rest will be a little easier.

BENT-OVER ROW

It's a great move for building a big upper back, but the technique can be tricky. Here's how to do it right

» Often overlooked by many, the bent-over row is a vital move that will help forge a strong upper back. If you spend most of your workout time on your chest and neglect your back then this can lead to a muscular imbalance that brings your shoulders forward. Not only does this not look good, it also increases your risk of injury.

That's why the bent-over row is so important. It works the opposite muscle group to the bench press, specifically the powerhouse muscles of the upper back – traps, lats, rhomboids and rear deltoids – and the biceps also assist the lift, while your abs must be involved to keep your torso straight and stable.

Target

- Upper back
- Biceps
- Core
- Lats

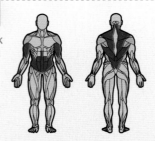

How to do it

- Grip the bar with an overhand grip just wider than shoulder-width apart.

- Stand with your core braced, your back straight and your shoulder blades retracted.

- Bend your knees slightly and lean forward from the hips, not the waist.

- Pull the bar up to your lower sternum, fully retracting your shoulder blades to allow the bar to come up to your chest, then lower the bar slowly to the start.

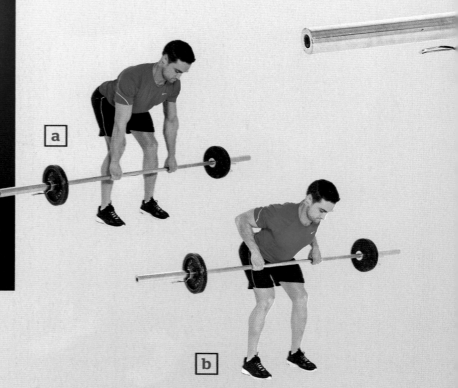

a

b

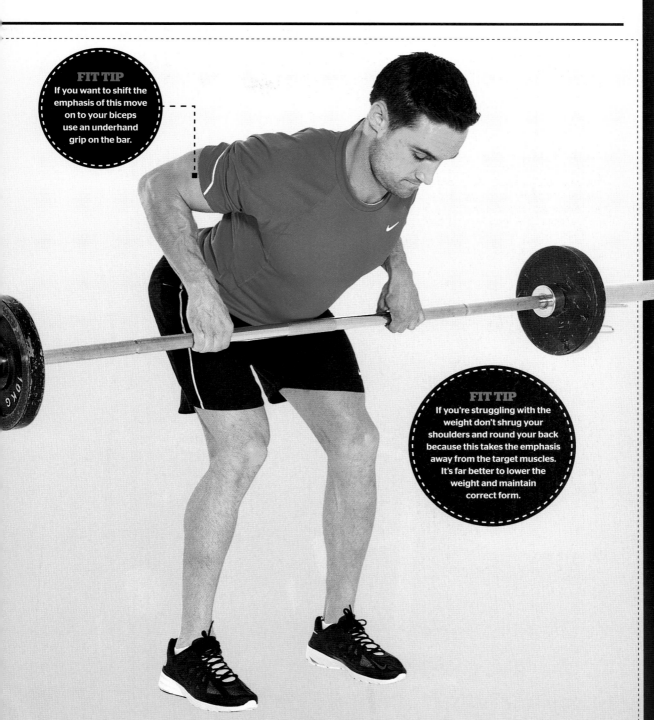

FIT TIP
If you want to shift the emphasis of this move on to your biceps use an underhand grip on the bar.

FIT TIP
If you're struggling with the weight don't shrug your shoulders and round your back because this takes the emphasis away from the target muscles. It's far better to lower the weight and maintain correct form.

TRICEPS DIP

Build big arms with this surprisingly tough bodyweight move

>> When wanting to build big arms it may be tempting to favour biceps moves over those exercises that focus on the triceps, but this isn't the right approach. That's because the triceps make up about two-thirds of your upper arm musculature, so you can't afford to ignore this muscle if you want to add size. Dips are one of the best moves to target all three parts of the triceps muscle, as well as being great for working the lower chest, shoulders and your core, which you must keep tight to prevent your lower body swinging.

Target

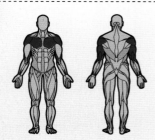

- Triceps
- Chest
- Shoulders

How to do it

- Grip parallel bars, keeping your body upright.

- With your elbows pointing straight back, lower your body as far down as you can comfortably go without stressing your shoulders.

- Keep your core braced and don't swing your legs for momentum.

- Push back up strongly to return to the start.

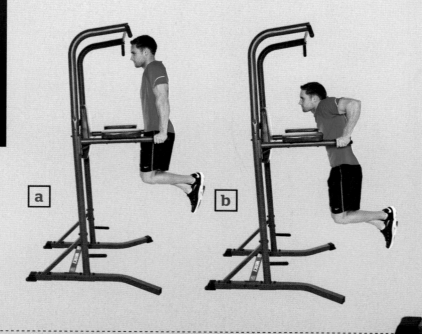

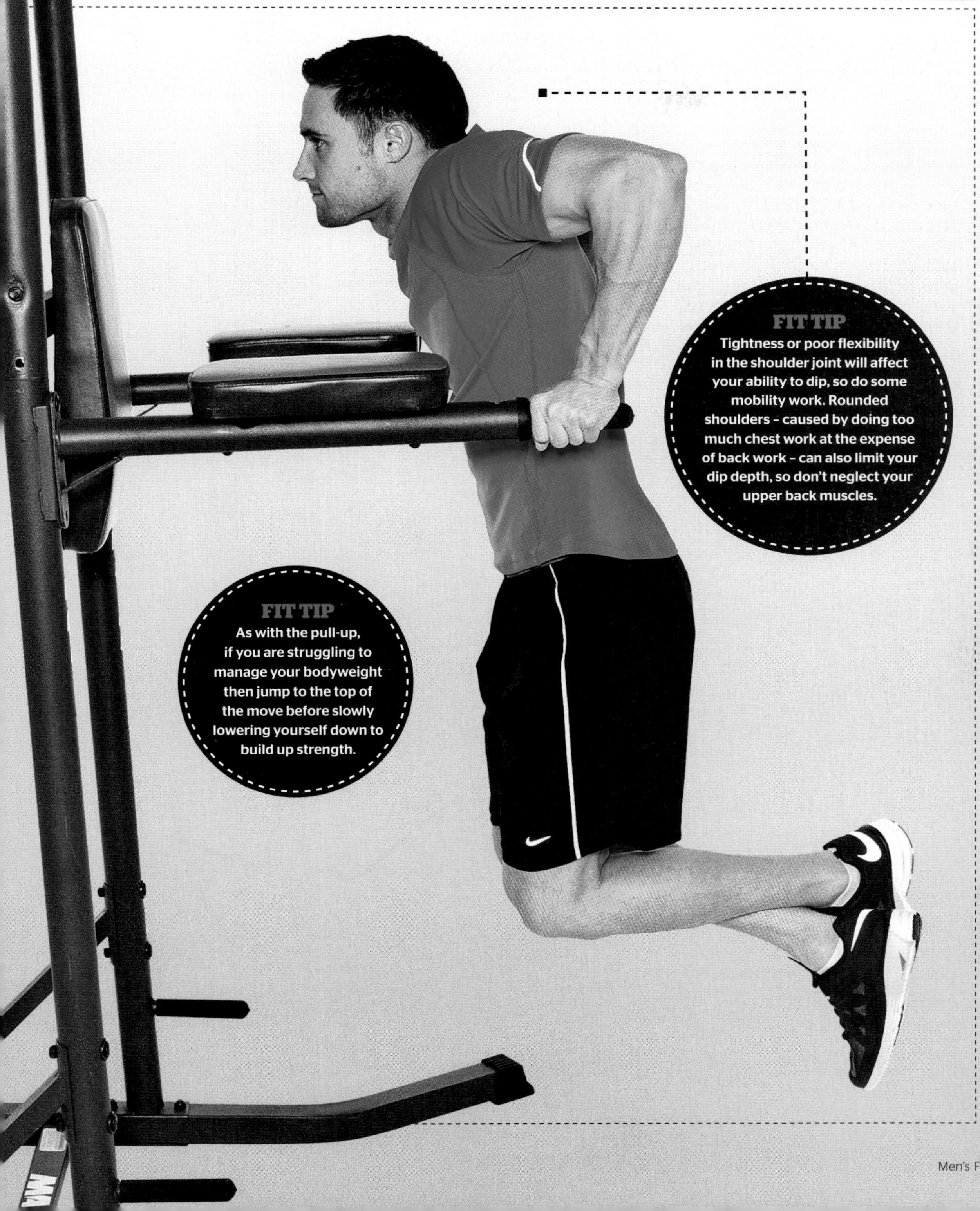

FIT TIP

Tightness or poor flexibility in the shoulder joint will affect your ability to dip, so do some mobility work. Rounded shoulders – caused by doing too much chest work at the expense of back work – can also limit your dip depth, so don't neglect your upper back muscles.

FIT TIP

As with the pull-up, if you are struggling to manage your bodyweight then jump to the top of the move before slowly lowering yourself down to build up strength.

CLEAN

This power-building move builds strength and stability from top to toe

>> The clean involves almost all your major muscle groups, forcing them to work together so you can efficiently move the bar from the floor to shoulder-height as quickly as possible. That makes it a high-risk move so start with a light barbell and master the correct form before adding additional weight. But big risk equals big rewards, and get this exercise right and you'll and build explosive power that has a great crossover to many sports and everyday activities.

Target

I Whole body

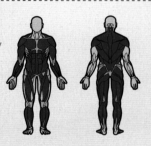

How to do it

● Stand with your shins touching the bar and feet shoulder-width apart.

● Squat down and hold the bar with an overhand grip.

● Keeping your core braced, your chest up and a natural arch in your back, lift the bar off the ground by driving up through your heels.

● Once the bar reaches your hips, rise up on tiptoes, shrug your shoulders powerfully and pull the bar up higher, leading with your elbows.

● As the bar travels towards shoulder height, squat back down under the bar and rotate your elbows forward so you catch it on your fingers and the front of your shoulders.

● Reverse the move back to the start.

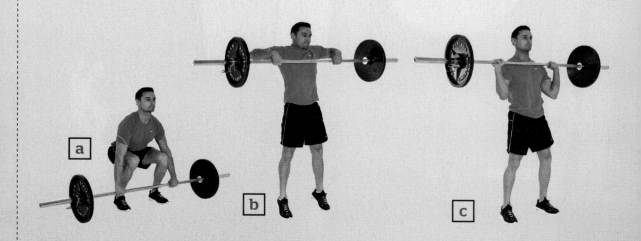

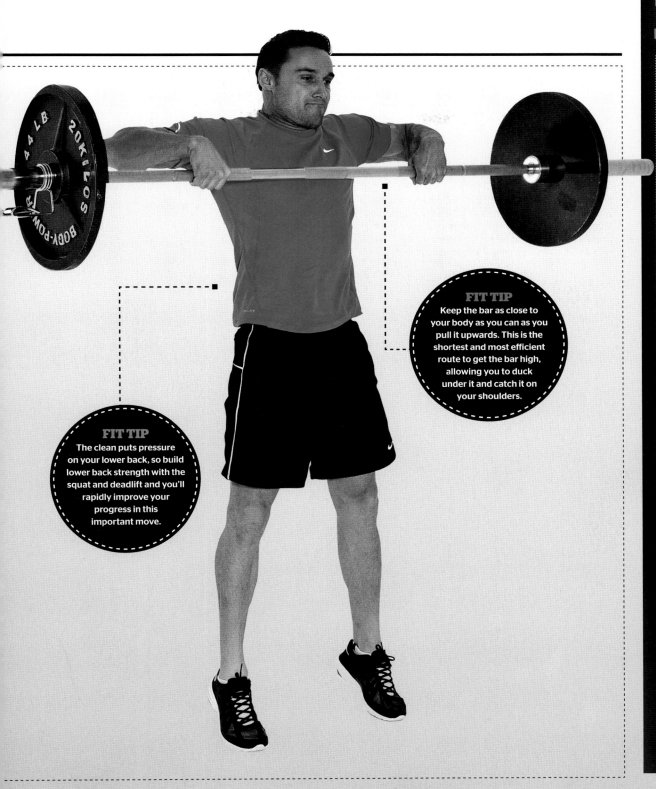

FIT TIP
Keep the bar as close to your body as you can as you pull it upwards. This is the shortest and most efficient route to get the bar high, allowing you to duck under it and catch it on your shoulders.

FIT TIP
The clean puts pressure on your lower back, so build lower back strength with the squat and deadlift and you'll rapidly improve your progress in this important move.

SNATCH

Funny name, serious move: the snatch is a highly effective whole-body muscle-building lift

This Olympic lift not only builds muscle but also flexibility and co-ordination. Targeting your entire posterior chain – all the muscles down the back of your body, from neck to calves – the snatch is more commonly associated with powerlifters than regular gym-goers. But that doesn't mean you shouldn't use it to improve your explosive power, strength, speed and core stability. Besides, many sports mimic its movement pattern in some form – for example, lifting a rugby player in the lineout. As with all big lifts, you need to ensure you set up correctly and focus your mind completely on the lift to get it right.

Target

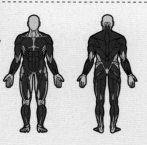

▌Whole body

How to do it

● Stand with feet hip-width apart with your shins touching the bar.

● Squat down, keeping a natural arch in your back and your chest out, and grip the bar with hands wider than shoulder-width apart.

● Push down through your heels and straighten your legs to lift the bar off the ground, keeping it as close to your legs as possible.

● As soon as it reaches your thighs, pull your shoulders back and bring the bar up hard and fast, 'flipping' the bar over and onto your fingers while getting your body under the bar by dropping into a squat position.

● Finish the movement by standing up out of the squat with your legs fully straightened, holding the bar directly above your head with your arms extended.

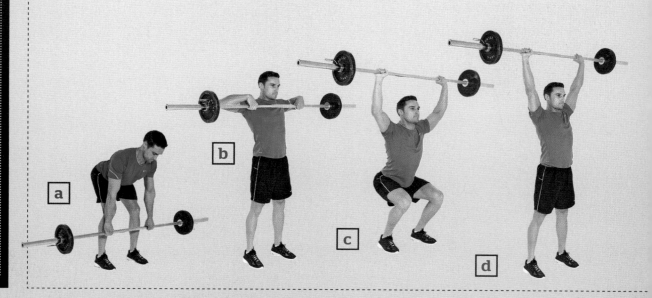

a

b

c

d

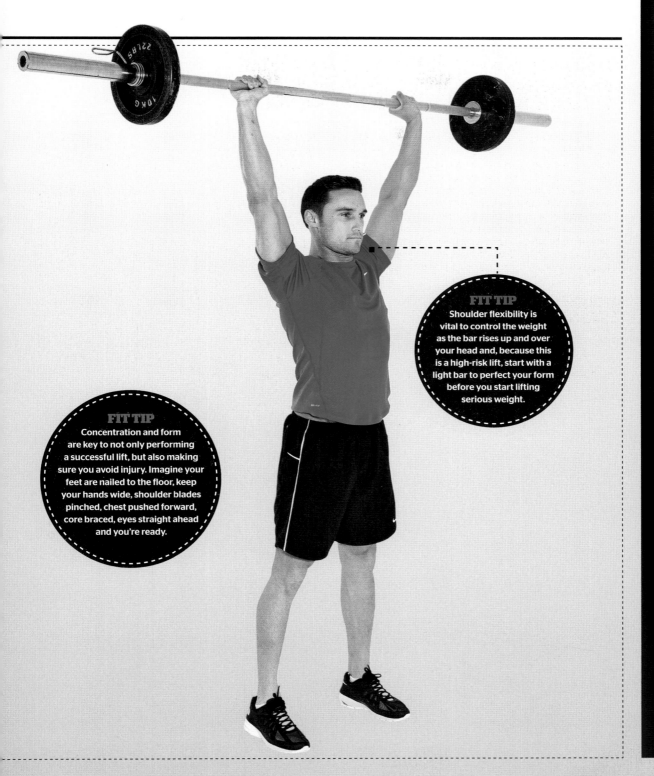

FIT TIP
Shoulder flexibility is vital to control the weight as the bar rises up and over your head and, because this is a high-risk lift, start with a light bar to perfect your form before you start lifting serious weight.

FIT TIP
Concentration and form are key to not only performing a successful lift, but also making sure you avoid injury. Imagine your feet are nailed to the floor, keep your hands wide, shoulder blades pinched, chest pushed forward, core braced, eyes straight ahead and you're ready.

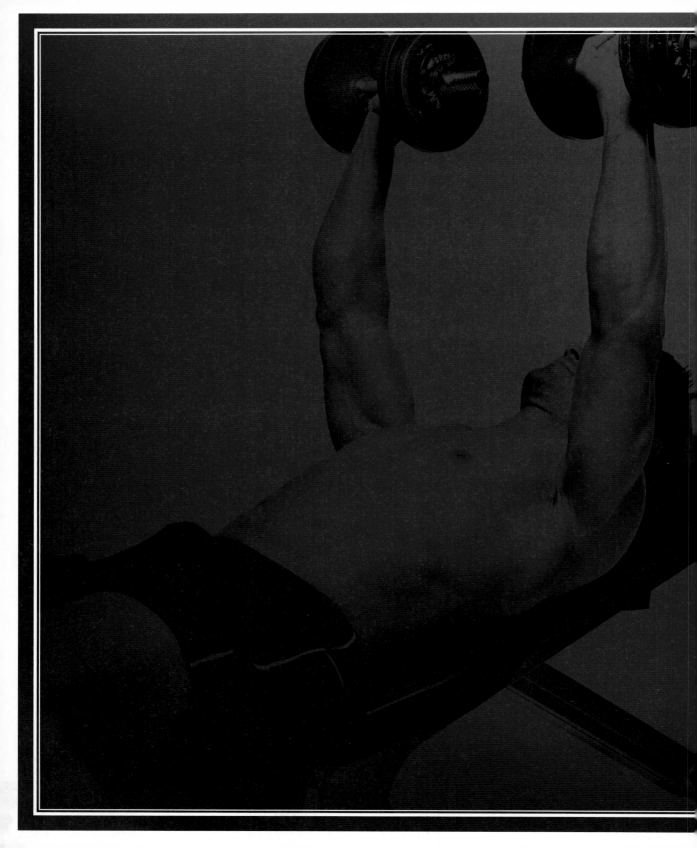

VARY YOUR EXERCISES

CONTENTS

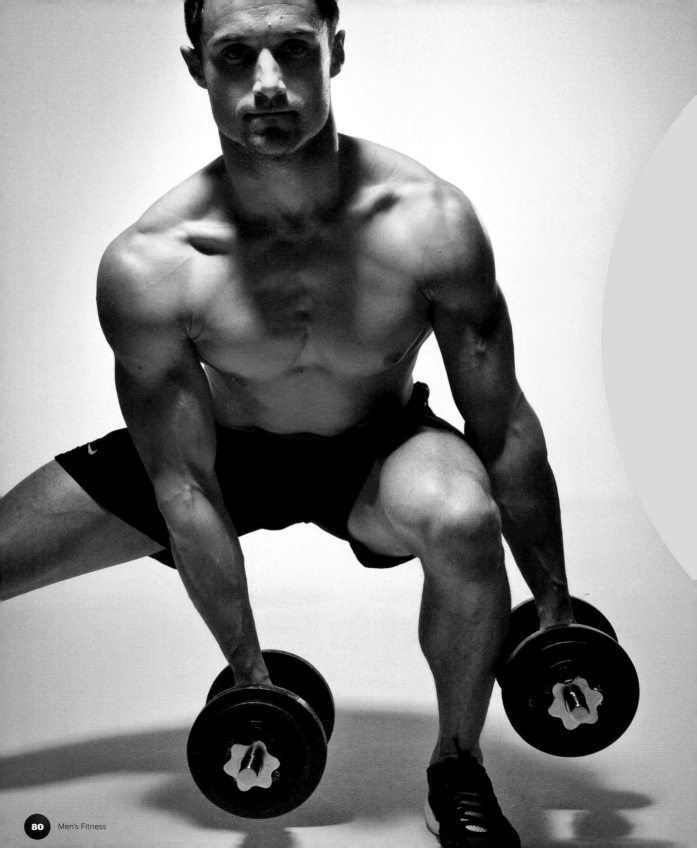

RULE FOUR | VARY YOUR EXERCISES

Why should I vary my exercises?

Variety isn't just the spice of life: it's also the only way to keep your muscles growing

>> If you are new to weight lifting putting on muscle is easy at first. But after a while you may notice that your gains begin to slow down or even plateau completely.

That's because your body very quickly adapts to the new stresses it has been exposed to in the gym. Your muscles become more efficient at performing the moves you do most often, which means that they don't have to work as hard to do the same amount of work. In short, performing the same exact workout week in, week out isn't an effective strategy to keep building muscle.

Plus, doing the same session is really, really boring. You'll never add muscle if you don't go to the gym because your bored with doing the same old session.

Shake things up
Luckily, there's a very simple solution to this problem. If you want to keep your muscles growing, you must keep them guessing. And the that means you need to regularly shake things up by introducing new exercises that will 'shock' your muscles into growth because they are unfamiliar with these new moves or variations and the new mechanics they involve.

Fresh look
Sometimes this will mean introducing a completely new move that hits the same muscles. At other times it will simply mean tweaking a move slightly, by say changing your hand position, the angle of the bench, your grip on the bar, or standing up instead of sitting down.

In this chapter you find an array of new exercises, all twists on the classic ten compound lifts of the previous chapter - plus a close look at some of the key isolation moves - that you can introduce into your training programme to keep your mind focused and your muscles working hard.

SQUAT VARIATIONS

These three twists on the classic squat can lead to big lower-body gains

DUMB-BELL SQUAT

»» WHY DO IT? If you struggle to maintain good form with a barbell, performing squats with dumb-bells can help you learn to do the move safely.

How to do it

- Stand tall with feet shoulder-width apart, holding a dumb-bell in each hand by your sides.

- With you core braced and a natural arch in your back, squat down until your thighs are at least parallel to the floor, keeping your knees in line with your toes.

- Push back up through your heels to complete the move.

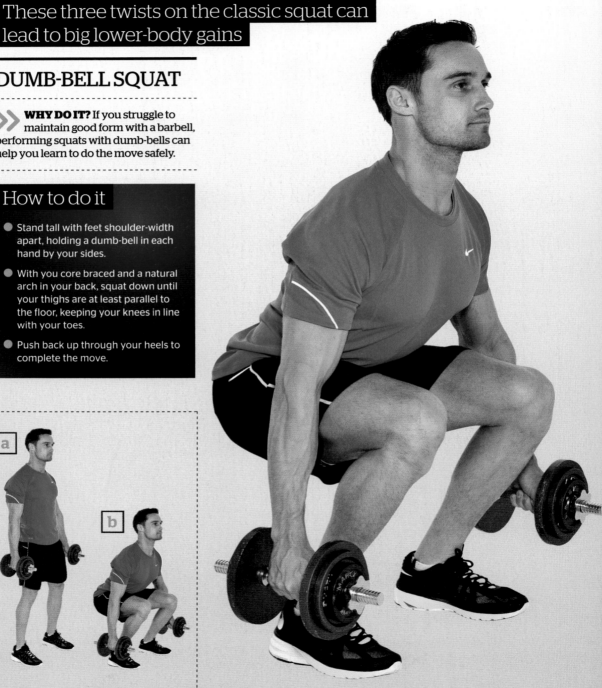

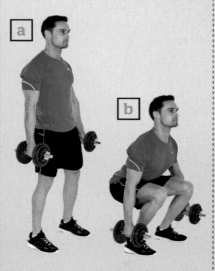

HACK SQUAT

>> **WHY DO IT?** Holding the bar behind your body forces you to keep your torso upright to manage the weight, and so improves your ability to perform normal squats correctly.

How to do it

- Standing in front of a barbell, squat down and pick up the bar using an overhand grip. Your feet should be shoulder-width apart.

- Squat down until your thighs are at least parallel to the floor, keeping your knees in line with your toes.

- Drive back up through your heels.

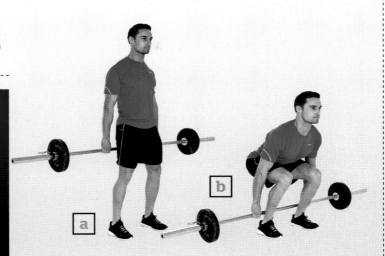

ZERCHER SQUAT

>> **WHY DO IT?** Holding the bar in the crook of your elbows takes the stress off your back, while forcing your core muscles to work hard to stabilise your upper body.

How to do it

- Take a barbell in the crook of your elbows, keeping your core braced and a natural arch in your back. Feet should be shoulder-width apart.

- Squat down until your thighs are at least parallel to the floor, keeping your knees in line with your toes.

- Drive back up through your heels.

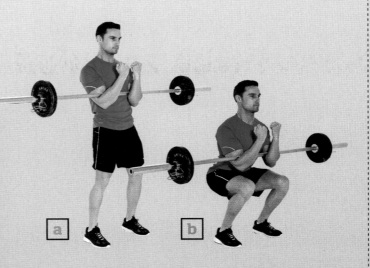

BENCH PRESS VARIATIONS

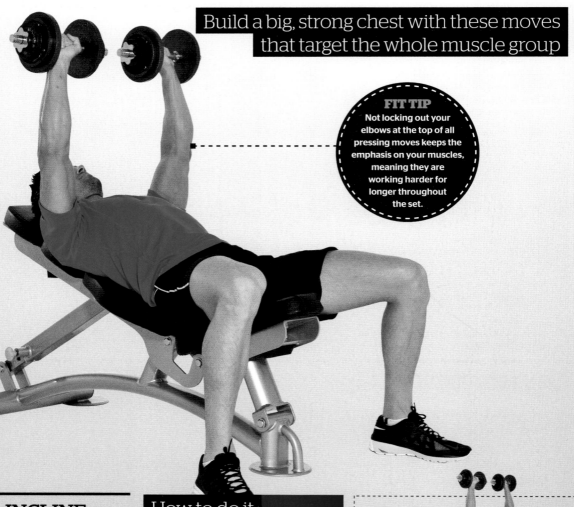

Build a big, strong chest with these moves that target the whole muscle group

FIT TIP
Not locking out your elbows at the top of all pressing moves keeps the emphasis on your muscles, meaning they are working harder for longer throughout the set.

INCLINE DUMB-BELL PRESS

>> **WHY DO IT?**
Tilting the bench upwards places the focus on your upper chest, as well as the front of your shoulders and triceps, while using dumb-bells allows for a greater range of motion.

How to do it

- Lie on a bench set at a 30-45° angle holding a dumb-bell in each hand at shoulder height.

- Keep your feet flat on the floor and back against the bench.

- Press the weight above your head but don't lock out your elbows.

- Slowly lower the weight back down to your chest.

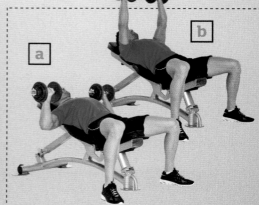

INCLINE DUMB-BELL FLYE

WHY DO IT? This move isolates your chest muscles – by taking your triceps out of the equation – so all the work has to be done by your chest.

How to do it

- Lie on an incline bench holding a dumb-bell in each hand directly above your chest.
- Ensure your head and shoulders are supported on the bench and your feet are flat on the floor.
- Keeping a slight bend in your elbows, slowly lower the weights as far to the side as comfortable. Squeeze your chest muscles to reverse the movement.

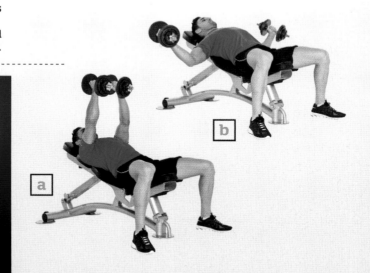

DECLINE BENCH PRESS

WHY DO IT? This variation targets the lower part of your chest.

How to do it

- Set a bench on a 30-45° decline. If you gym doesn't have a decline bench then place a secure box or Reebok Deck under one end.
- Hold a bar using an overhand grip, hands shoulder-width apart.
- Slowly lower it down to your chest, flaring your elbows out to the side to keep the emphasis on your chest.
- Push back strongly to the start position, but don't lock out at the top.

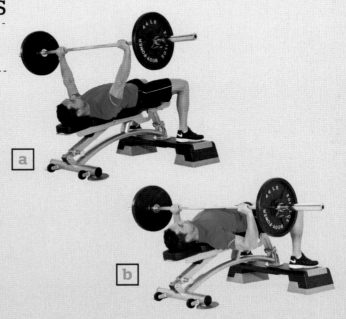

DEADLIFT VARIATIONS

A strong back makes all other lifts easier. Here's how to build one

GOOD MORNING

WHY DO IT? This move works the erector spinae along with hamstrings and glutes. It's a great move, but maintain perfect form throughout to prevent injury and start with a light bar.

How to do it

- Stand tall with a light barbell resting across the top of your shoulders. Hold the bar just outside your shoulders.

- Brace your core, retract your shoulder blades and maintain a natural arch in your back throughout the move.

- Feet should be between hip- and shoulder-width apart with a slight bend in your knees.

- Bend forward slowly from the hips, not the waist, and lean forward as far is your hamstrings allow, but not past horizontal.

- Return back to the start.

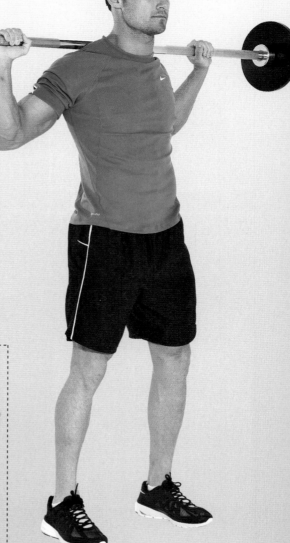

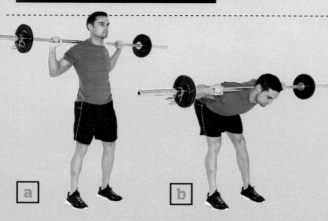

SUMO DEADLIFT

>> **WHY DO IT?** By taking a wider stance you recruit your glutes and stretch your adductors.

How to do it

- Stand behind the bar with your feet wider than shoulder-width apart and your toes pointing outwards.

- Squat down and grip the bar with your hands shoulder-width apart.

- Keeping a natural arch in your back, drive with your legs and push your hips forward to lift the bar until you are standing upright.

- Reverse the movement to return the bar to the floor.

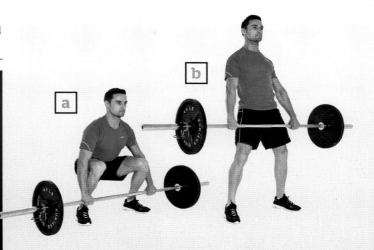

BARBELL SUITCASE DEADLIFT

>> **WHY DO IT?** Because the weight is on only one side, your abs have to work hard to keep your torso upright and stable. You are also going to be hitting your glutes, obliques and lats as you work each side of the body. It will improve your grip strength too.

How to do it

- Place a barbell on your left side. Crouch down into a deadlift position and grab the middle of the bar with your left hand.

- Brace your core, keep a natural arch in your back and drive with your legs to deadlift the bar up to thigh height while keeping it parallel to the floor.

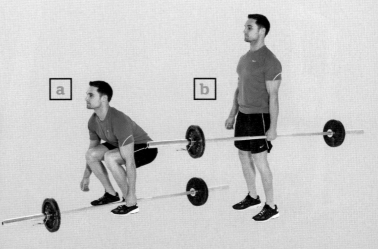

PULL-UP VARIATIONS

Master these classic back moves for a big, strong, and balanced upper body

CHIN-UP

» **WHY DO IT?** Using an underhand grip shifts the focus to your biceps, making it easier while still taxing all the major muscles of your upper back.

How to do it

- Grab the bar with an underhand grip with your hands closer than shoulder-width apart.

- Start from a dead hang with your arms fully extended.

- Pull yourself up by squeezing your lats together.

- Once your chin is higher than your hands pause briefly, before slowly lowering yourself back to the start.

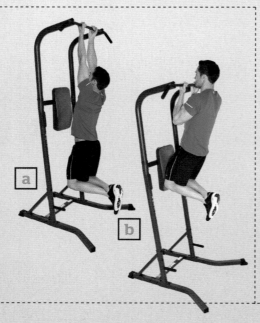

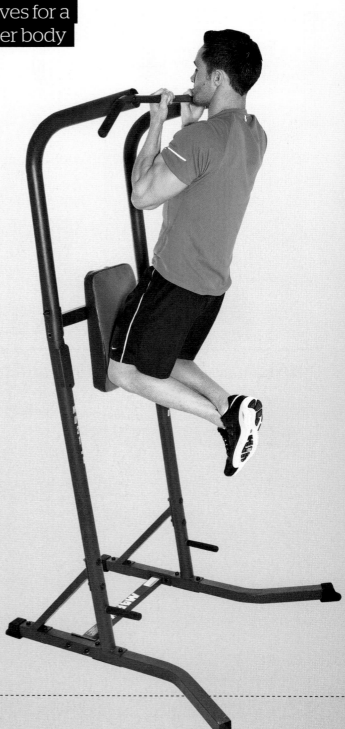

LAT PULL-DOWN

≫ WHY DO IT? The machine lets you easily adjust the resistance, so you can lift lighter or heavier than your bodyweight.

How to do it

- Sit on the seat and take an overhand, wide-grip on the bar.
- Look forward, retract your shoulder blades and keep your torso upright.
- Pull the bar down in front of you until it reaches your upper chest. Don't lean back to aid the movement.
- Squeeze your lats at the bottom of the move and return the bar slowly to the top.

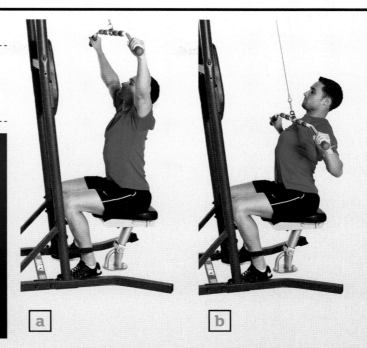

DUMB-BELL PULLOVER

≫ WHY DO IT? Although a single-joint move, this exercise works a large number of muscles, specifically lats, chest and triceps.

How to do it

- Lie on a bench with shoulders and head supported, feet flat on floor.
- Hold a single dumb-bell with both hands over your chest and engage your core.
- Slowly lower the weight behind your head, keeping a slight bend in your elbows. Don't arch your back.
- Pull your arms back over your head to the start.

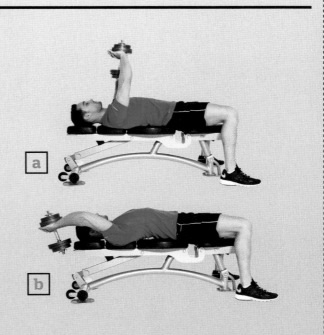

LUNGE VARIATIONS

Work your legs, glutes and lower back with these twists on the classic li

ROMANIAN DEADLIFT

» **WHY DO IT?** This is one of the best moves for building muscle mass on the backs of your legs. Perfect form is vital to protect your lower back from injury. Always lean forward, slowly, from your hips and not your waist and control the bar slowly down your shins.

How to do it

● Hold a barbell with an overhand grip just outside your hips. Stand with feet shoulder-width apart, shoulder blades retracted, torso upright, core braced and a natural arch in your back.

● Lean forward from the hips and slowly lower bar down your shins until you feel a stretch in your hamstrings.

● Push your hips forward to reverse move back to start.

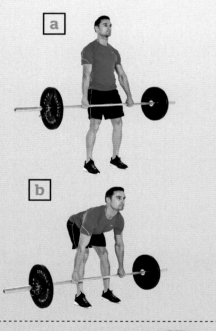

a

b

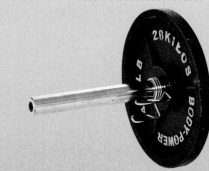

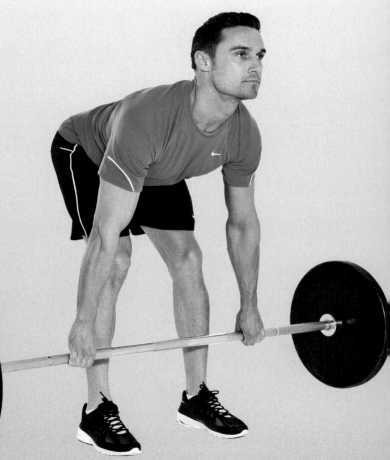

GYM BALL LEG CURL

>> **WHY DO IT?** Although it uses only your own bodyweight, this tough move hits your hamstrings hard.

How to do it

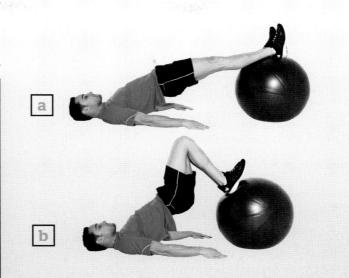

- Lie with head, shoulders and upper back on a gym mat with your feet together on top of a gym ball. Your body should form a straight line from head to heels.

- With your back straight, raise your hips and use your heels to drag the ball toward you.

- Pause briefly at the top of the move before slowly returning to the start.

DUMB-BELL LATERAL LUNGE

>> **WHY DO IT?** Ignoring your inner thigh muscles can lead to muscular imbalances and injury but if you strengthen them with this move you'll improve all in lower-body lifts.

How to do it

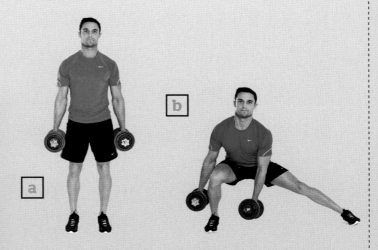

- Stand tall with feet close together, holding a dumb-bell in each hand.

- Keeping your core braced and head looking forward, take a big step to the side with your right leg and lower your body down so your right knee is in line with your toes.

- Push back off your right leg and repeat the other side.

SHOULDER PRESS VARIATIONS

Build broad shoulders to create that V-shape torso

PUSH PRESS

>> **WHY DO IT?** Using your legs to initiate the move enables you to lift more weight and prevent poor form at the start of each rep.

How to do it

- Stand tall with a barbell across your upper chest. Hold the bar with an overhand grip just wider than shoulder-width apart.

- Keeping your core braced, bend your knees slightly before standing back up while at the same time pressing the bar directly overhead by straightening your arms. Don't lock out your elbows.

- Slowly return the bar back down to the start.

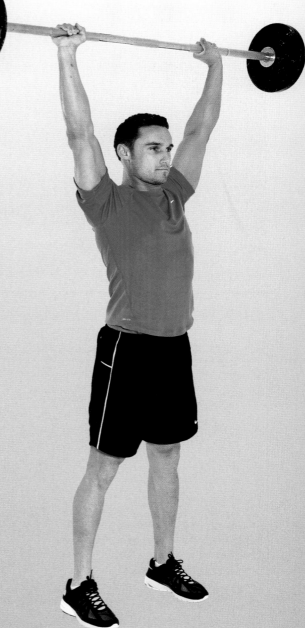

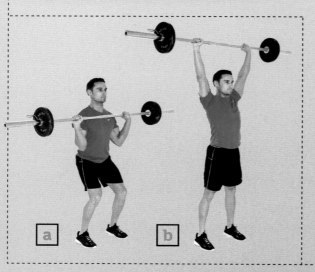

a b

ARNOLD PRESS

>> **WHY DO IT?** This variation combines a pressing action with a rotational one, hitting your deltoids from several angles.

How to do it

- Sit on an upright bench with a dumb-bell in each hand with palms facing you.

- Keep your feet flat on the floor, core braced, back against the bench and head looking forward.

- Press the weights up, rotating your palms so that you finish with arms extended and palms facing away.

- Reverse the movement back down to the start.

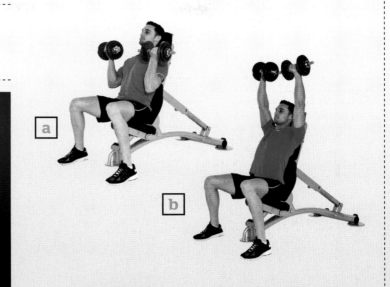

BARBELL CUBAN PRESS

>> **WHY DO IT?** It works the rotator cuff, the stabilising muscles of the shoulder joint, which will allow you to lift heavier on other shoulder moves.

How to do it

- Hold a light barbell with an overhand grip at thigh height.

- Raise the bar until it's at shoulder height.

- Rotate your arms so that your hands point up, keeping your biceps horizontal.

- Press the bar directly overhead before reversing the movement back to the start.

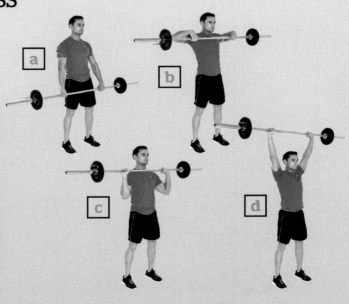

BENT-OVER ROW VARIATIONS

Hit your back and biceps with these tweaks on the row

ONE-ARM ROW

»» WHY DO IT? Focusing on one arm at a time prevents you from relying too much on your stronger arm to do most of the work. This ensures you achieve more balanced gains.

How to do it

- Place your left knee and left hand flat on a bench, with your right leg out to the side. Hold a dumb-bell in your right hand.

- With a natural arch in your back and core braced, lift the weight up towards your side, leading with your elbow.

- Slowly return the weight back to the start and repeat both sides.

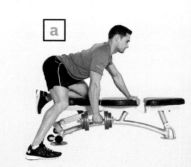

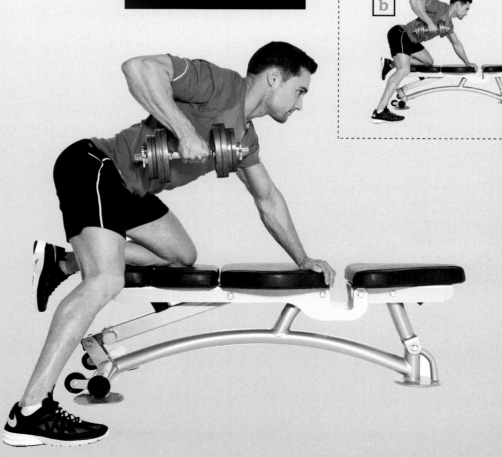

INVERTED ROW

>> **WHY DO IT?** As well as working your back muscles and biceps, this puts more emphasis on your core and lats and helps correct bad posture.

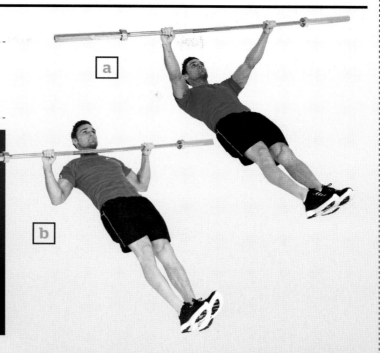

How to do it

- Set a Smith machine bar at about chest height. Hold the bar using an overhand grip, with hands just wider than shoulder-width apart, and with your feet on the floor.

- Hang until your arms are fully extended then, keeping your hips in line with your torso, pull your body up to the bar until you touch it with your sternum.

- Lower yourself slowly.

SEATED CABLE ROW

>> **WHY DO IT?** Hitting your back muscles while seated focuses your efforts on the target muscle groups and lets you lift heavier weights.

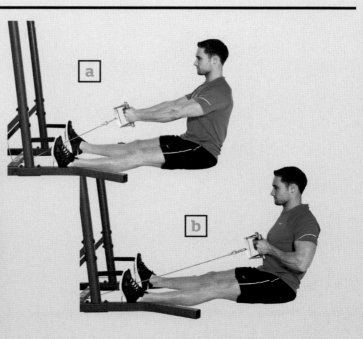

How to do it

- Sit with a flat back and a slight bend in your knees. Using a neutral grip, take hold of a double-D handle attached to the bottom pulley of a cable machine.

- Ensure that there is tension in the cable before you begin.

- Pull the handle into your sternum, keeping your torso still. Squeeze your shoulder blades together and return slowly to the start.

TRICEPS DIP VARIATIONS

Build big and powerful arms with these triceps-targeting moves

CLOSE-GRIP BENCH PRESS

» WHY DO IT?
Bringing your hands closer together transfers the focus of this move away from the chest and on to the triceps – making it a great move for building big upper arms.

How to do it

- Lie flat on a bench and hold a barbell using an overhand grip, about a fist-width apart, with arms fully extended.

- Keep your body flat on the bench, and your feet flat on the floor.

- Lower the bar slowly, keeping your elbows close your sides.

- Push up powerfully, but don't lock out your elbows.

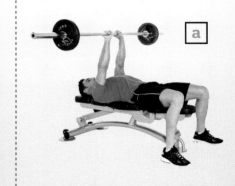

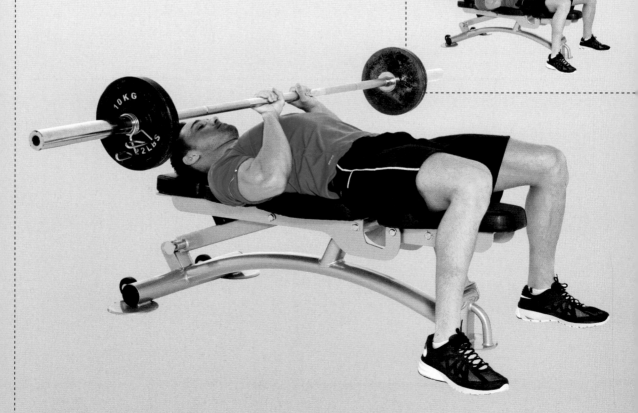

MEDICINE BALL PRESS-UP

»» WHY DO IT? This press-up variation places greater emphasis on the triceps, while the instability of the ball forces your core to work overtime to keep your body rigid.

How to do it

- Start in a press-up position but with your hands either side of a medicine ball, rather than flat on the floor.

- Keeping your body in a straight line from head to heels, lower your chest down until it touches the ball before powering back up strongly.

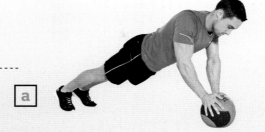
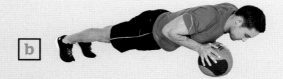

DIAMOND PRESS-UP

»» WHY DO IT? Having your hands close together shifts the focus away from the chest towards your triceps, making this a great any-time and any-place move for upper-arm mass.

How to do it

- Start in a press-up position but with your hands close together so that opposite thumbs and index fingers touch to form a diamond shape.

- Keeping your body in a straight line from head to heels, lower your chest down as far as you can, then press back up strongly.

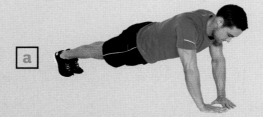
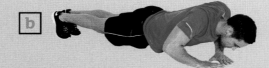

CLEAN VARIATIONS

Build total body strength with these complementary clean moves

FRONT SQUAT

» WHY DO IT?
Resting the bar on the front of your shoulders targets your quads while protecting the lower back. With the bar in front, it's also impossible to lean forward, so you get a deeper range of motion.

How to do it

● Rest the bar on the front of your shoulders, gripping it with your hands crossed in front of you, your elbows pointing forward and feet shoulder-width apart.

● Maintain a natural arch in your back and keep your core braced.

● Squat down until your thighs are at least parallel to the floor.

● Push back up through your heels.

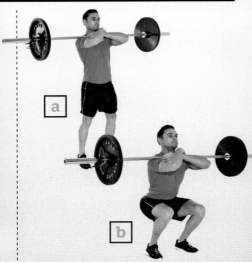

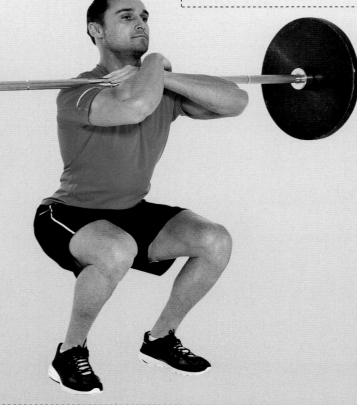

HANG CLEAN

» **WHY DO IT?** Starting with the bar at mid thigh height helps you master the move safely, but as your legs aren't so involved, you'll have to lift lighter.

How to do it

- Hold a barbell with an overhand grip, feet shoulder width apart.

- Rise onto your tiptoes, shrug your shoulders and pull the bar up, leading with your elbows.

- Once the bar reaches your shoulders, squat under it and rotate your elbows forward so you catch the bar on your fingers and the front of your shoulders.

- Reverse back to the start position.

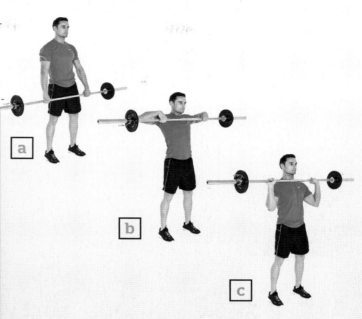

KETTLEBELL CLEAN

WHY DO IT? This move will increase your strength and stability as well as improve your form on the clean.

How to do it

- Hold a kettlebell between your legs, with back straight and chest up.

- Bend your knees and push the kettlebell back between your legs. Stand up and drive your arm forward while pushing your hips forwards to propel the weight to above head height then flip it over onto the front of your shoulder.

- Reverse back to the start.

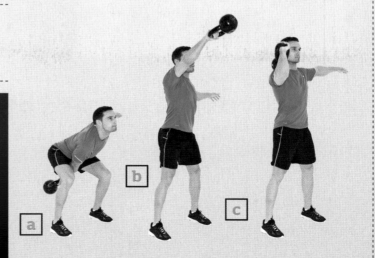

SNATCH VARIATIONS

Improve your strength, power and co-ordination with these supplementary snatch moves

KETTLEBELL SNATCH

» WHY DO IT? This move works each side of the body independently and it also engages your core throughout to keep your torso upright. In addition it will help improve your form for the snatch, enabling you to lift heavier without the risk of injury.

How to do it

- Hold the kettlebell in one hand and swing it up by snapping your hips forward. Keep your core engaged and a natural arch in your back.
- As the kettlebell passes waist height pull your shoulder back, then punch your arm forward as it passes shoulder height.
- Catch the kettlebell on your forearm at full extension.

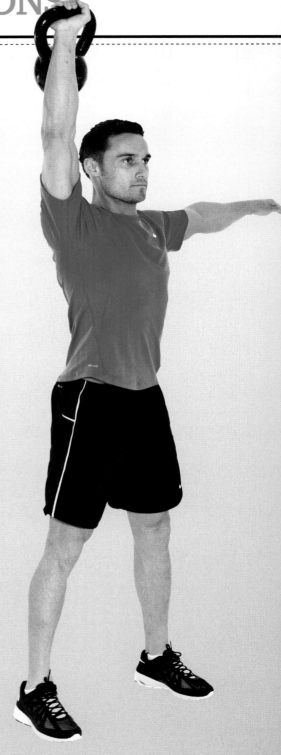

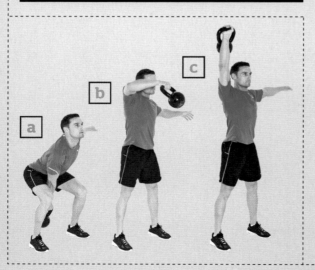

UPRIGHT ROW

>> **WHY DO IT?** Although this move mainly works your traps and shoulders, getting a strong upper back helps with the 'shrugging' part of the main snatch lift, letting you generate the power to lift the bar over your head.

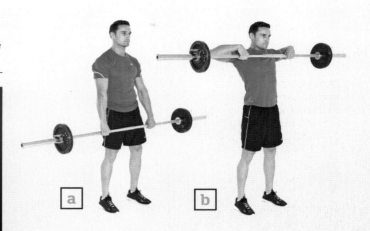

How to do it

- Stand tall holding a barbell with an overhand grip slightly narrower than shoulder width.
- Shrug the bar up towards your chin, leading with your elbows pointing to the ceiling.
- Slowly lower the bar back to the start position.

OVERHEAD SQUAT

>> **WHY DO IT?** This tough twist on the classic squat is the final part of the snatch lift, and getting better at this will benefit a host of other moves.

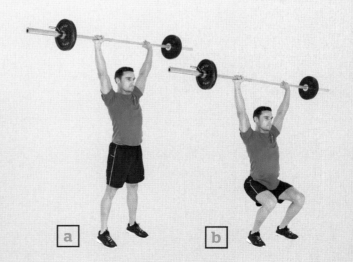

How to do it

- Hold a light barbell overhead using a wide overhand grip.
- Your feet should be shoulder-width apart, your core braced, with a natural arch in your back.
- Squat down as far as you can without allowing your back to arch forward.
- Drive back up through your heels to complete the move.

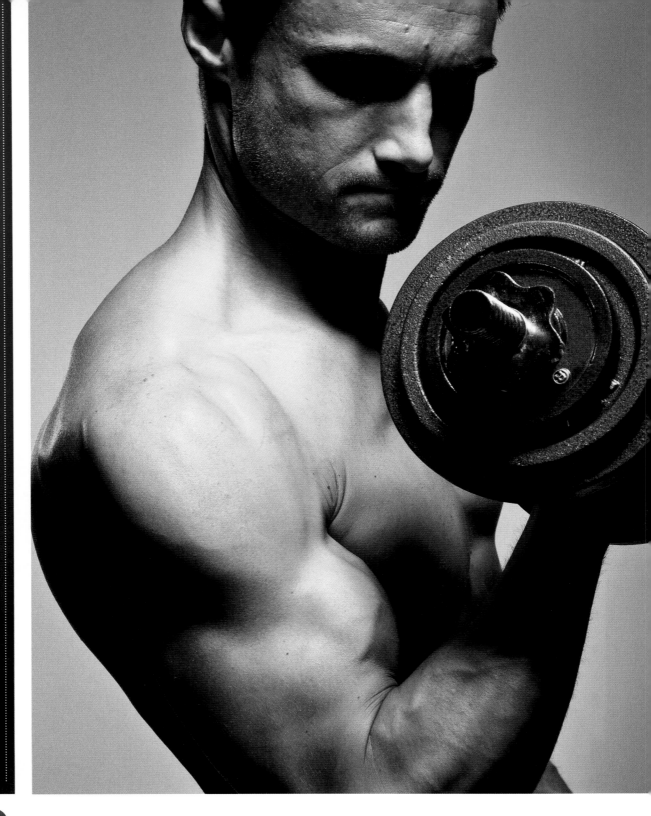

Splendid isolation

Target specific muscles with isolation moves for quicker and more impressive growth

>> Compound lifts should certainly form the backbone of your training regime as they recruit the most muscle groups. But this doesn't mean you need to consign all isolation moves to the scrap heap completely.

To remind you, isolation moves are those lifts that cause movement at only one joint, while compound moves are multi-joint exercises that work multiple muscle groups (see page 54 for the major compound exercises).

Consequently, isolation lifts work less well at quickly adding a lot of muscle mass across your body, but they are ideal when you want to target a specific muscle to try and coax extra growth.

One way these single-joint moves can be used successfully is as a 'finisher', that is an exercise performed at the end of a workout to really fatigue the target muscles. Take for example an arms workout (see page 136 for how to construct a workout) where the majority of the session is built around compound lifts, such as chin-ups, pull-ups, bent-over rows and close-grip bench presses.

After all of that you will be tired, but your biceps and triceps may still have a little energy left in them. So to break down even more muscle fibres and encourage greater muscle growth, you could finish the session with sets of isolation lifts, such as EZ-bar biceps curls and lying triceps extensions. Unlike compound moves, where your risk of injury is higher if you're tired, these isolation moves can be performed safely.

Extra push

Putting in that little extra effort can completely exhaust those target muscles, and so force your body to grow them back bigger and stronger.

Over the next few pages we'll highlight some of the best isolation exercises for each of your major muscle groups, allowing you to safely but effectively push your muscles harder to promote faster gains. What's not to like?

BICEPS

EZ-BAR BICEPS CURL

Blitz your biceps with this classic isolation move

WHY DO IT? A biceps curl can also be performed with a barbell or with a dumb-bell in each hand, but using an EZ-bar, which has a zigzagged middle, allows you to turn your hands inwards slightly. This takes some of the strain off your wrists and allows the focus of the weight to be solely on your biceps, forcing them to work harder throughout the move.

How to do it

- Stand with your shoulders back and feet close together and hold an EZ-bar using an underhand grip with your hands just outside your hips.

- Keeping your elbows tucked in to your sides, curl the bar up towards your chest, stopping just before your forearms reach vertical.

- Lower back slowly to the start.

- Avoid rocking back and forth to generate momentum, which takes the emphasis away from the biceps.

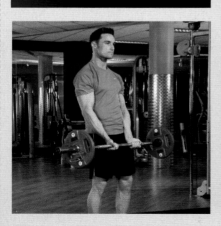

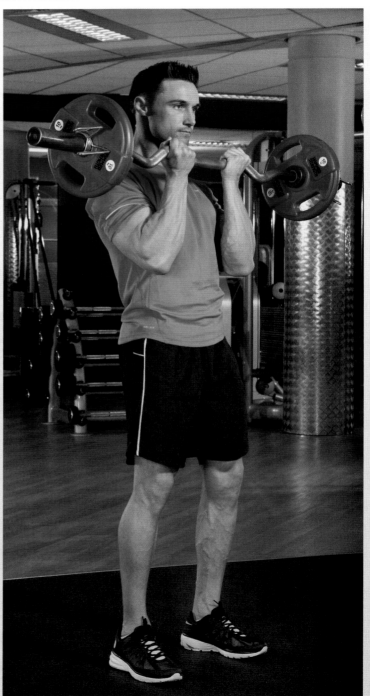

ONE-ARM PREACHER CURL

Work each arm separately for growth

>> WHY DO IT? Resting your upper arm on a preacher bench stops you from using momentum and forces your biceps to do all the work. Training each arm individually also prevents your dominant arm carrying more of the load, resulting in balanced growth. Fully straighten your arm at the bottom of the move, and squeeze your biceps at the top, for maximum muscle gains.

How to do it

- Hold a dumb-bell in one hand and rest that upper arm against the preacher bench.

- Curl the weight up until your forearm is vertical.

- Squeeze your biceps at the top of the move before lowering slowly back to the start.

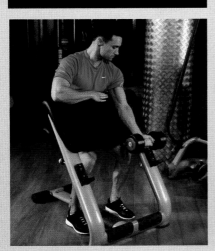

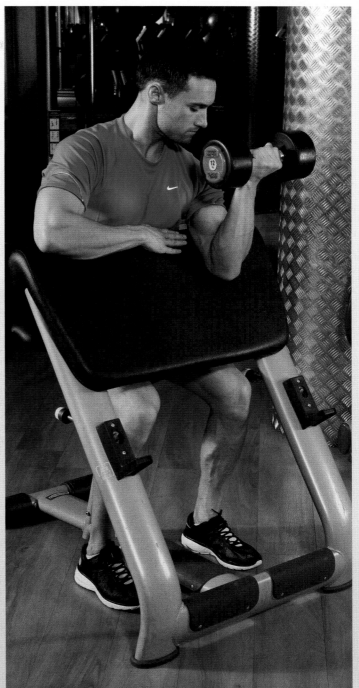

TRICEPS

LYING TRICEPS EXTENSION

Build upper-arm mass by isolating your powerful triceps

>> WHY DO IT? It isolates your triceps, forcing them to work hard throughout the move to control the weight down then raise it back up. Start by using a light weight because you need to manage the weight safely as you lower it towards your head. Otherwise you may find out why this move is also known as the nose-breaker or skull-crusher.

How to do it

- Lie flat on a bench, holding an EZ-bar above you with straight arms.

- Slowly lower the bar towards the top of your head by bending your elbows, which should stay pointing directly to the ceiling.

- Without arching your back, slowly return the bar to the start position by straightening your arms.

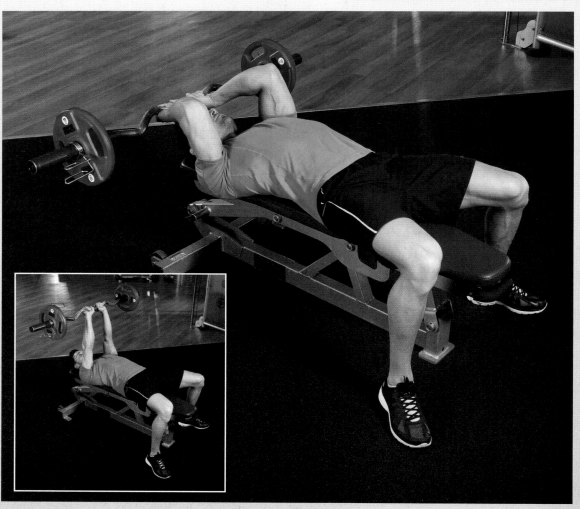

TRICEPS PRESS DOWN

Work your triceps with this cable move

» **WHY DO IT?** The advantage of using a cable machine is that there is resistance throughout the whole move, forcing your triceps to work hard to manage the weight on the way up as well as on the way down. Keep your elbows close to your sides so the emphasis stays on your triceps.

How to do it

- Stand tall at a cable machine with a double rope handle or straight bar handle attached at head height.

- Keeping your elbows tucked in, press the handle down without leaning forward.

- Squeeze your triceps at the bottom of the move before slowly returning back to the start.

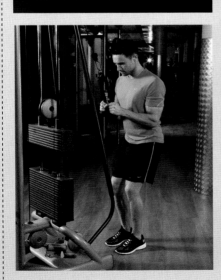

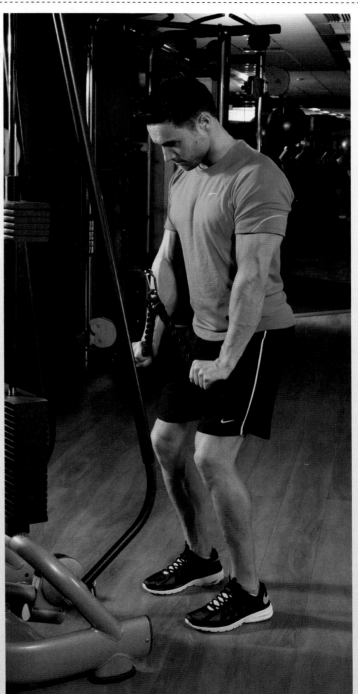

CHEST AND SHOULDERS

CABLE CROSSOVER

Craft a big chest with this powerful move

» WHY DO IT? Truly isolating your chest muscles can be hard because your arms and shoulders nearly always get in on the act. But using cables, rather than dumb-bells, as resistance ensures that there is constant tension throughout the move, which forces your chest to work hard throughout.

How to do it

- Stand in the middle of a cable machine with your feet together holding a D-handle attachment in each hand, and with the cable set above shoulder height.

- Keeping a natural arch in your back, your core braced and upper body still, bring your hands down in an arc to meet in front of your chest.

- Pause briefly and squeeze your chest muscles before returning slowly, and under full control of the weight, back to the start position.

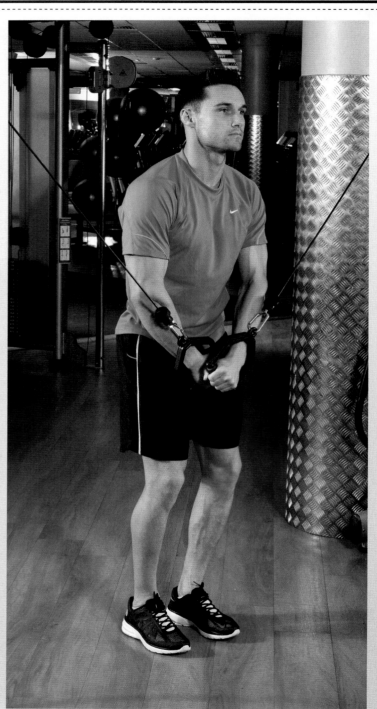

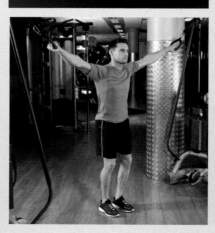

LATERAL RAISE

>> **WHY DO IT?** The lateral raise is effective at isolating the deltoids, the three muscles that make up the shoulders. However, because the shoulder joint is the most delicate in the body, keep the weights light and control the move from start to finish.

How to do it

- Stand tall with your core braced and your feet slightly apart. Hold a light dumb-bell in each hand with palms facing one another.

- Keeping a slight bend in your elbows, raise the weights out to the sides to shoulder height using your muscles and not momentum. Pause at the top, then slowly lower.

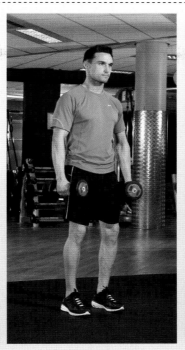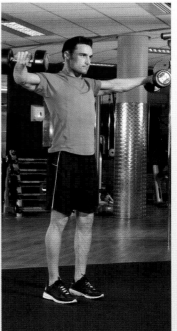

SHRUG

>> **WHY DO IT?** Shrugs have a limited range of motion, which means that you can use heavy dumb-bells to build big and strong traps that help create desirable wide shoulders.

How to do it

- Stand tall holding a heavy dumb-bell in each hand, keeping your core braced and a natural arch in your back.

- Shrug your shoulders towards your ears, keeping your arms straight, and the dumb-bells by your sides.

- Hold for a second at the top position before slowly lowering the weight back down.

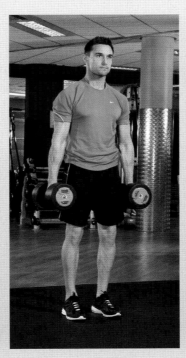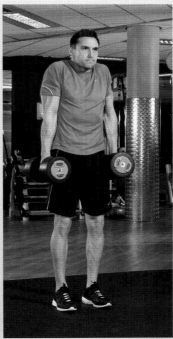

LEGS

SEATED LEG EXTENSION

Isolate your quads with this machine move

>> **WHY DO IT?** The best way to isolate your powerful quad muscles is to use a leg extension machine, rather than freeweights. This machine provides stability for your upper body and the movement path is fixed, meaning all your energy can be focused on working the quads to the max.

How to do it

- Sit on the machine, following its instructions to position yourself correctly and safely.
- Ensure that your knees are aligned with the lever to reduce the risk of injury and that your shins are against the padded bar.
- Keeping your back against the seat and your core braced, extend your knees to straighten your legs and raise the bar up.
- Return slowly to the start.

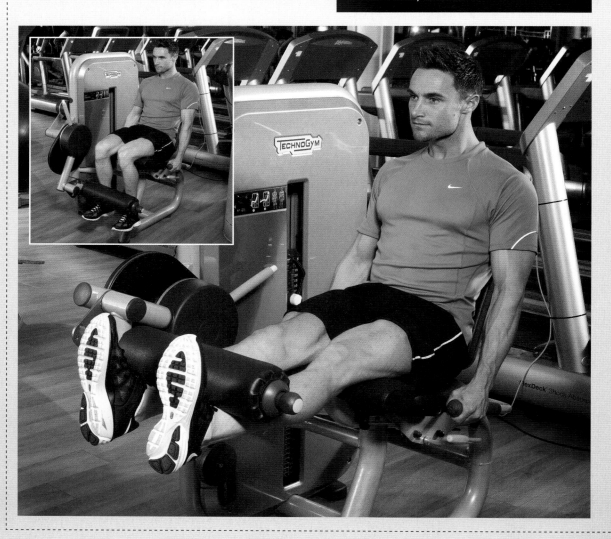

SEATED HAMSTRING CURL

>> **WHY DO IT?** The same principles apply here: the machine provides the stability and fixed movement pattern so you can work your hamstrings to total fatigue.

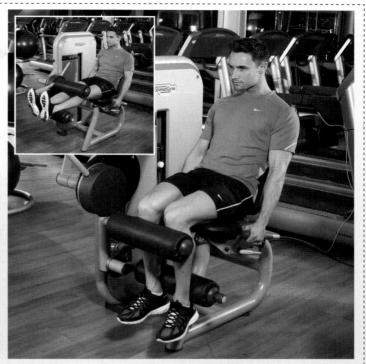

How to do it

- Position yourself safely on a leg curl machine, following its instructions, with the top bar sitting comfortably below your knees and the bottom one flat against the bottom your calves.

- Slowly contract your hamstrings to bring the padded bar against your calves towards you.

- Return slowly to the start position.

SEATED CALF RAISE

>> Training the calves can be hard using freeweights because you need to go really heavy to fatigue these muscles that are used to hard work – they're responsible for every step you take each day. Instead use a machine to fully isolate your calves without the injury risk that comes with using a very heavy barbell or set of dumb-bells.

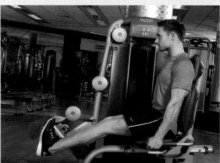

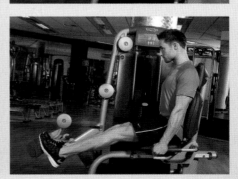

How to do it

- Sit on a seated calf raise machine, following its instructions to position yourself correctly and safely.

- Place the top of your toes on the platform. There should be a slight bend in your knees in this start position.

- Push your toes away to raise the weight.

- Pause briefly before returning back to the start, ensuring you go through the full range of motion to really work this hard-to-grow muscle.

FIX YOUR WEAK SPOTS

Proud of your prominent biceps and big chest? They might be impressive, but if you don't work all your muscles you'll end up with an unbalanced body. Here's how to make all-over gains

 1 ### MISSING MUSCLE
ROTATOR CUFF

This muscle doesn't need to be big but it does need to be strong, so you neglect it at your peril. A weak rotator cuff can lead to injury and put you out of action for months. But if you improve your shoulder stability by working this critical shoulder stabiliser you'll ward off injury and increase your power output in lifts, such as the shoulder press, and in sports such as volleyball, tennis and baseball.

Include a set of internal rotation exercises before every training or sports session to both warm up and strengthen the rotator cuff.

KEY MOVE
Barbell Cuban press (see page 93)

WHEN?
Do this at the start of your shoulder workout with a light weight to thoroughly warm up this delicate muscle group.

 2 ### MISSING MUSCLE
FOREARMS

Guaranteed to help with your grip, strong forearms can also help the overall development of your arms and assist with many heavy compound lifts, such as pull-ups and deadlifts. So if you want to build bigger biceps, triceps and shoulders your grip strength is incredibly important. Without a strong grip not only will you severely limit your ability to lift heavy, but you'll also increase your risk of injury to your shoulders.

KEY MOVE
Collar grip (see page 62)

WHEN?
Do this after your heavy sessions when your grip is already fatigued to work the forearm muscles even harder.

 3 ## MISSING MUSCLE CALVES

Ask any gym-goer if they train their legs and they'll probably answer 'Of course!' with an offended look. Ask them how much of that time is spent on their calves, however, and the look is more likely to be one of embarrassment. The calves are the engine of the body, working tirelessly no matter what you're doing. Because of this they are classed as an endurance muscle and building these takes a two-pronged attack. Aim for some straight-leg calf raises for the calf, and a bent-knee version to hit the soleus, which is the deep-lying calf muscle that connects your knee to your foot. Go heavy – these muscles need stimulating.

KEY MOVE Seated calf raise (see page 111)

WHEN? Do this at the end of your leg session and aim for three sets of at least 12 reps.

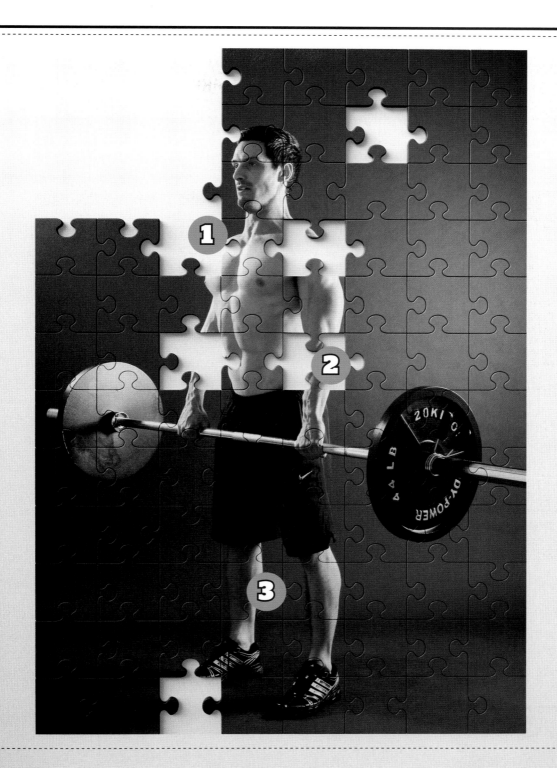

FIX YOUR WEAK SPOTS

4 MISSING MUSCLE
TRAPEZIUS

Your trapezius muscles, or traps – either side of your spine below your neck – are responsible for neck and shoulder strength, and working them can give you an impressively wide physique. They're activated by the shrugging motion and move your scapulae (shoulder blades) up, down and back. Exercises that mimic a shrug will strengthen your upper traps, while your lower traps work in conjunction with your lats to perform pull-ups and lat pull-downs. Traps are important to assist in developing other muscles, such as lats and rear deltoids. Include either dumb-bell or barbell shrugs in your back or shoulder workouts to develop these muscles.

KEY MOVE
Dumb-bell shrugs (see page 109)

WHEN?
At the end of your session perform three sets of eight to 12 reps with a heavy weight to target this powerful muscle.

5 MISSING MUSCLE
REAR DELTOID

This muscle – the back part of your shoulders – is key to achieving wide, strong and impressive upper body because big rear deltoids give width and mass to your upper back. You also need to train these, along with the rotators, to improve shoulder stability. Benches and other pressing exercises often place too much emphasis on the front deltoid so ignoring the rear part of this muscle group can cause imbalance and injury.

KEY MOVE
Bent-over lateral raise

HOW TO DO IT
Stand with your feet shoulder-width apart and a dumb-bell in each hand. Bend forward from the hips, with the weights at arm's length, palms facing each other, then raise the weights until they're in line with your shoulders. Slowly lower to the start. Do three sets of ten to 12 reps at the end of a shoulder workout.

6 MISSING MUSCLE
HAMSTRINGS

Underdeveloped hamstrings leave your legs weak and prone to injury but regular hamstring exercises and stretches will make these muscles strong and flexible, which in turn will prevent you pulling them when you're performing intense exercise such as sprinting. As your hamstrings are the muscles that help propel you forward, building bigger hamstrings will also help to increase your running speed .

KEY MOVE
Seated leg curl (See page 111)

WHEN?
Aim for three sets of eight reps after lunges to isolate your hamstrings. And after hitting your legs with squats and deadlifts, finish off your leg routine with three sets of seated leg curls, with ten to 12 reps in each set.

7 MISSING MUSCLE
GLUTES

Building your glutes has far more than cosmetic benefits. When working properly, your glutes are the most powerful group of muscles in the body. They're so crucial to movement that other muscle groups are equipped to assist in or even take over some of their roles if they're not up to the job. This substitution of movement often leads to loss of muscle mass, pain and ultimately injury, so it's vital to train them. Do so by including squats, lunges and step-ups.

KEY MOVE
One-leg glute raise

HOW TO DO IT
Lie on your back with arms by your side. Keep one leg straight and bend the other so its foot is flat on floor. Push down on this foot to raise your glutes. Keep your core braced. Hold, then lower to the start. Do three sets of ten to 12 reps for each leg.

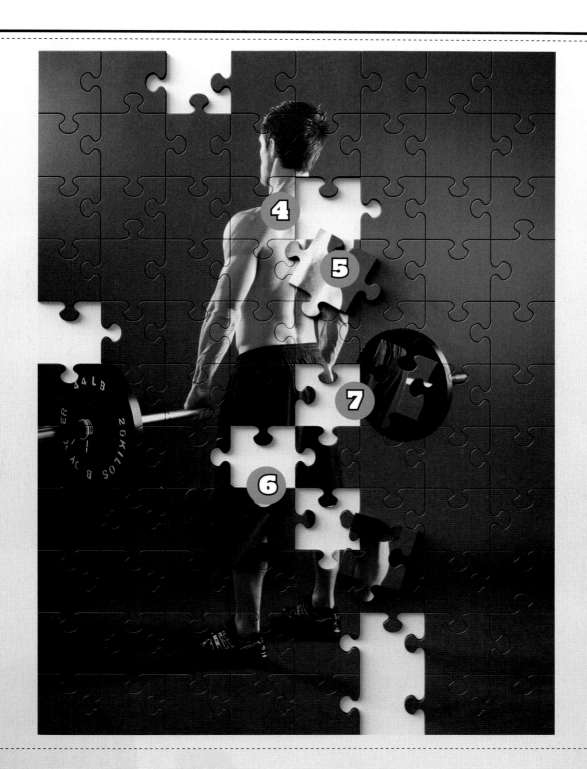

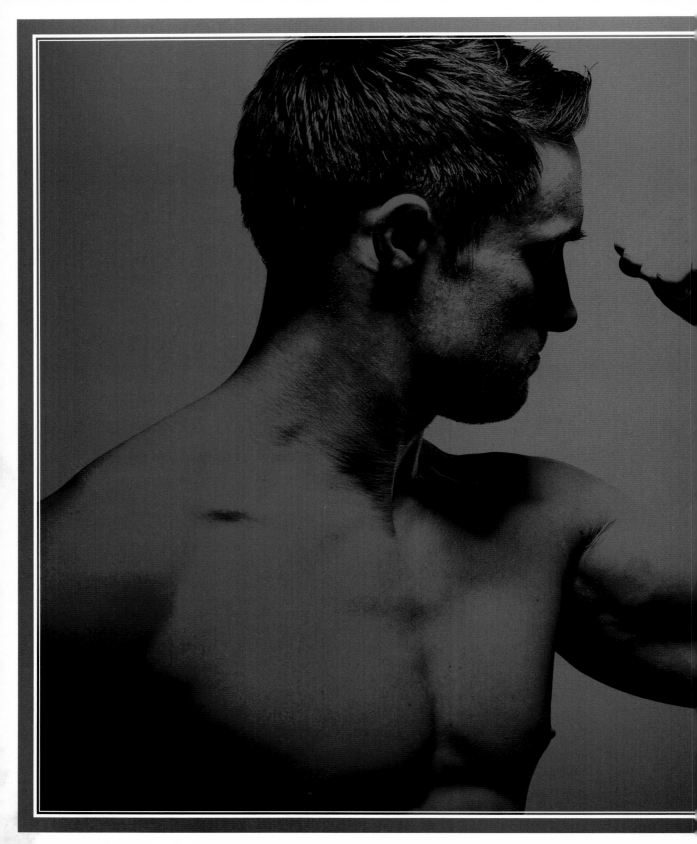

CHANGE THE VARIABLES

CONTENTS

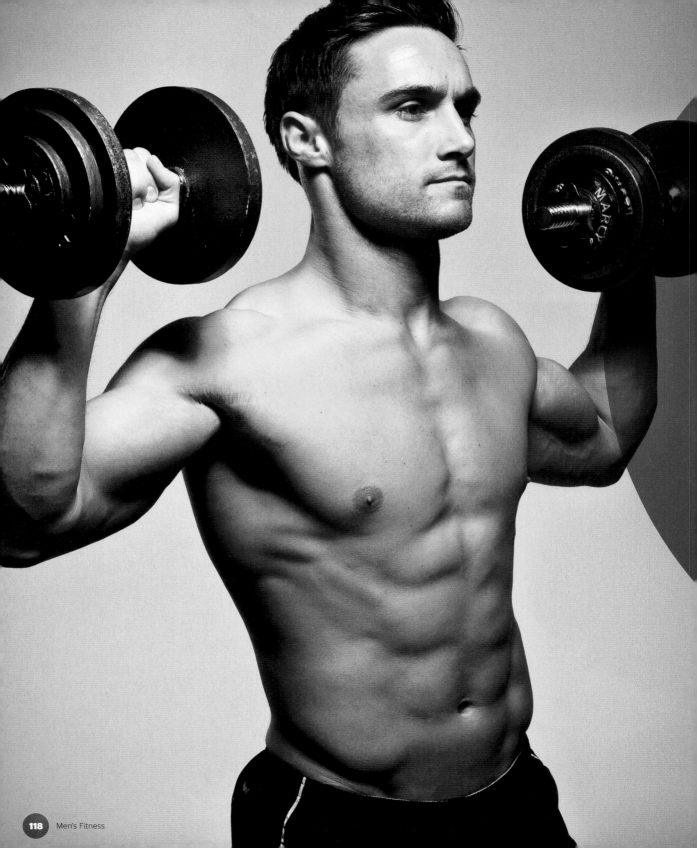

Why do you need to change the variables of your workout?

The elements that make up a workout and why you should mix them up to see your muscles grow

» Now you know the main compound and isolation exercises and how to perform them correctly, it's time to put your newfound knowledge into action and actually start building some muscle.

There are many types of workout you can do, and we'll take a closer look at some of the most effective options in chapter six. First, let's take a look at the key components of every workout and why you need to keep changing them.

The basics

A workout is made up of a number of different elements or variables:

Exercise selection The lifts you perform in any given workout.
Reps The number of times you perform a move without stopping for rest.
Sets The number of times you perform a certain number of reps.
Weight The amount of resistance you lift for each rep of each set.
Tempo The speed at which you perform each rep.
Rest The amount of time you rest between sets and between exercises.

Make a change

The most obvious variable between workouts is exercise selection. This and the weight you lift are the most important variables to keep changing for continued muscle growth. But tweaking all the key variables can also have a big impact on your muscle-building progress.

This chapter explains everything you need to know from the basics – how to select the correct sets and reps range – to how periodisation (see page 122) can help you to add 20 per cent to any lift in as little as nine weeks. It also covers everything in between, such as how often you should train, how fast you should lift and how long you should rest between exercises.

SETS AND REPS

If you don't know how many sets and reps you should be performing you'll never build muscle. Here are the basics of every workout

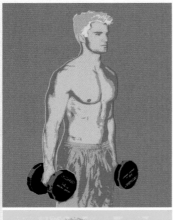
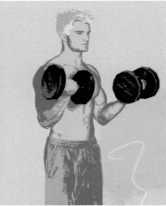
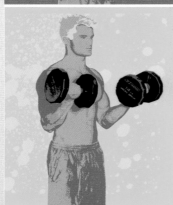
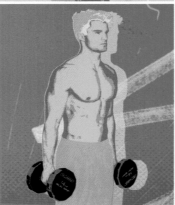
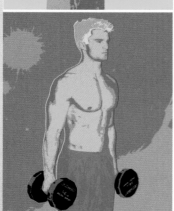
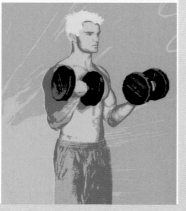

>> Sets and reps are the bread and butter of your workout. As soon as you lift a weight, even if it's only once, you've completed a rep – and a set. But doing one lift on its own is not the best way to build muscle.

Instead you need to lift a weight a certain number of times, rest for a given amount of time, then repeat this process a certain number of times.

The most effective sets and reps range for building muscle is three to four sets of eight to 12 reps of a given move. That's because this approach subjects your muscles to enough resistance and time under tension to ignite the muscle-building response.

To workout which weight you should be lifting you need to know your one-rep max, or the maximum amount of weight you can lift for a single repetition of any move.

Knowing this is important because percentages of this number determines the weight you should be lifting for each rep, depending on your training aim. Here's what you need to know.

At a glance
Reps and sets

REPS
An abbreviation of repetition, one rep is the completion of a given exercise from start to finish. To build muscle you need to perform between eight and 12 reps per set.

SETS
A set is a given number of reps performed consecutively without rest. Three to four sets of eight to 12 reps is the most effective way to increase muscle mass.

Picking the right rep range

Performing the appropriate number of reps per set at the right weight is critical to achieving your goals

1-5 REPS

TRAINING AIM Increase in your muscle strength and power.
WEIGHT 85-100 per cent of one-rep max.
WHY? Low-rep sets of heavy weights build strength and power because they recruit and fatigue your fast-twitch muscle fibres. They're responsible for your muscles' explosiveness and this approach makes them grow back bigger. This rep range also improves the communication pathway between your brain and the muscle, helping it to react and contract faster and with more force.

6-7 REPS

TRAINING AIM Optimal compromise between an increase in muscle strength and size.
WEIGHT 78-83 per cent of one-rep max.
WHY? Sets in this rep range will still work your fast-twitch muscle fibres and improve the brain-muscle connection, but performing extra reps will also fatigue your muscles more thoroughly, resulting in improvements in strength and size.

8-12 REPS

TRAINING AIM Increase in your muscle mass and improved strength.
WEIGHT 70-77 per cent of one-rep max.
WHY? The most effective way to build muscle mass is for each set to last between 40 and 70 seconds. Sets of eight to 12 reps are the perfect rep range for this because the weight is heavy enough to fatigue the muscles thoroughly but still manageable for you to maintain correct form for the desired length of time.

13+ REPS

TRAINING AIM Increase in your muscle strength-endurance with some muscle-mass gains.
WEIGHT 60-69 per cent of one-rep max.
WHY? Using lighter weights combined with a higher rep range recruits, works and fatigues your slow-twitch fibres. Sets in this rep range improve the ability of these fibres to deal with lactic acid and the other waste products that accumulate during exercise. You will still see some muscle-mass gains, however, especially if you are new to weight training.

Rep ranges and weight percentages taken from *German Body Comp Program* by Charles Poliquin (charlespoliquin.com)

DIFFERENT TYPES OF REPS

In addition to normal reps, try these variations to keep your muscles guessing – and growing

FORCED REPS

Once your muscles fail and can no longer perform a single extra rep, a training partner or spotter can step in to help you force out a few extra ones to break down even more muscle tissue. They do this by helping you get past the 'sticking point' of a given exercise – for example the first half of a biceps curl – before you take over to finish the rep's full range of motion.

NEGATIVE REPS

Your muscles are stronger in the eccentric, or lowering, phase of a lift than in the concentric, or raising, stage. Negative reps take advantage of this strength by using a much heavier weight and starting at the 'top' position of a move and then lowering it as slowly as possible, ideally in more than four seconds. So, you might jump to the top of the pull-up position then slowly lower back to the start, or have a spotter help you lift a barbell to the top of a biceps curl then lower it slowly.

PARTIAL REPS

These reps only involve movement through a certain part of an exercise's normal full range of motion. This is typically the easiest part of each rep where heavier weights can be used.

PERIODISATION

Increasing the weight each week is a sure-fire recipe for success

>> Many fitness experts trip over themselves in their attempts to bring you the latest, cutting-edge fitness thinking. However, sometimes the best advice has been around for some time. About 2,000 years, in fact.

Varying the intensity of training over a series of cycles to avoid a plateau – a process known as 'periodisation' – became popular in the 20th century, but it was the ancient Greeks who first realised the benefits. Legend has it that the strongman Milo of Croton used a baby bull as his training tool of choice. As the calf grew, so too did the weight Milo had to lift.

His fellow ancient Greek Galen of Pergamum (AD129-c216), a writer, philosopher and physician to gladiators, also advocated planned training variation, believing that using various forms of exercises would maximise performance.

Repetitive strain

Periodisation may be well established but that doesn't mean it's common knowledge in most weights room. It's probably true to say that one of the most common mistakes made in the pursuit of new muscle is lifting the same weight and doing the same thing week in, week out. >

JARGON BUSTER
Periodisation

Structuring training into progressively more challenging phases to improve strength and gain muscle.

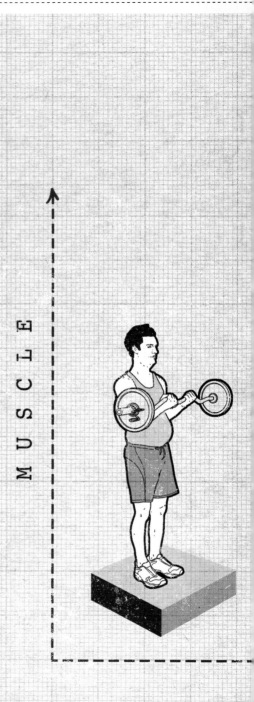

MUSCLE

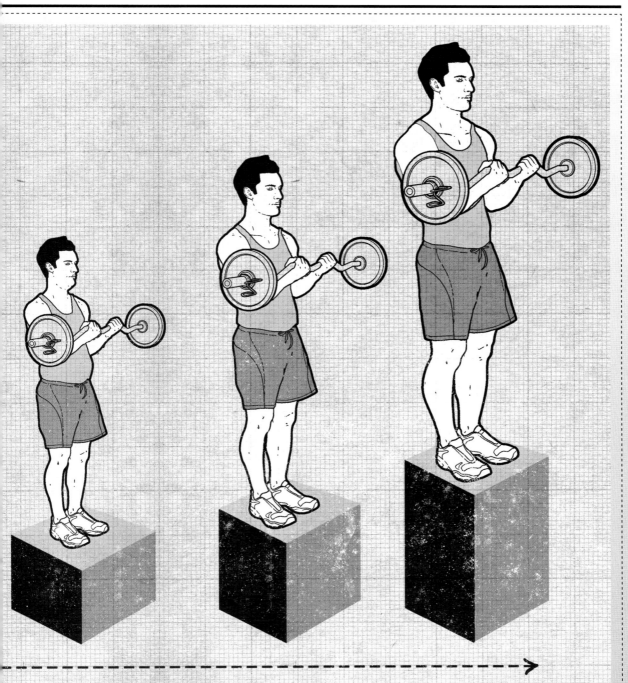

T I M E

PERIODISATION

Go down this route and keep doing the same thing at every workout session and, eventually you'll stop improving. But if you follow Milo's example and keep increasing the load you're lifting eventually you'll gain strength.

This phenomenon, known as general adaptation syndrome, is something periodisation seeks to exploit and sports scientists have explored.

A recent study at Texas A&M University took 92 weight-trained males divided them into four groups. The first group lifted sets of 79 per cent of their one-rep max, group two lifted 83 per cent and group three started at 79 per cent, but rose gradually to 92 per cent. Group four played badminton. After 16 weeks the members of group three, the only group that used periodisation, were stronger in both the bench press and squat than any of the other three groups.

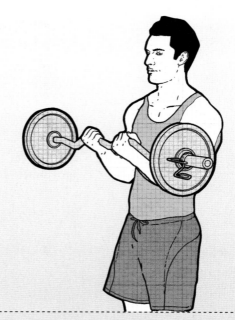

Real world benefits

Use periodisation to add 20 per cent to any exercise in nine weeks

This chart shows the progression you could make using periodisation over nine weeks if you are currently lifting 60kg for the bench press – but it's the structure of the progression, rather than the exercise, that's key. If you lift more or less than 60kg, adjust the starting weight but follow the same level of progression, making sure you don't add more than about 2.5 per cent each week.

Workout key
Workout A
Workout B
Workout C

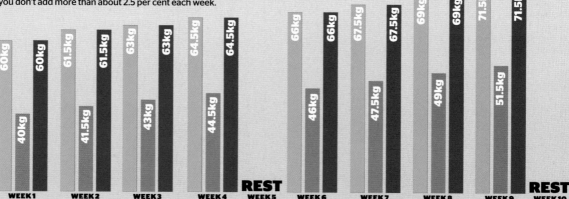

	Workout A	Workout B	Workout C
WEEK 1	60kg	40kg	60kg
WEEK 2	61.5kg	41.5kg	61.5kg
WEEK 3	63kg	43kg	63kg
WEEK 4	64.5kg	44.5kg	64.5kg
WEEK 5	REST		
WEEK 6	66kg	46kg	66kg
WEEK 7	67.5kg	47.5kg	67.5kg
WEEK 8	69kg	49kg	69kg
WEEK 9	71.5kg	51.5kg	71.5kg
WEEK 10	REST		

The scientific, and indeed mythical, evidence seems to support using periodisation, but you're still left with the question of how, specifically, you should apply it to your workouts. Taking a random approach just won't work.

Instead, decide what you want to achieve and use the training variables at your disposal to meet that goal.

If your goal is strength then use the correct reps and sets to achieve it. This might be four sets of five reps, so you progress on one variable, such as how much weight you lift. Aim to increase upper-body lifts by up to 2.5 per cent each week and lower-body lifts by up to five per cent.

A key part of periodisation is keeping a training log to track your progress because if you don't record what you do, you have no way of knowing whether you're increasing the stress you're placing on your body or whether you're improving.

Rest right

Another important aspect of periodisation is making sure you take rest or recovery weeks. It may seem like a waste of valuable workout time but without rest you won't make the same gains. You can use the same workouts for four to six weeks, improving week on week, but after that you may find you're not able to push on so it's a great idea to take a week off or a week of active recovery by doing half the volume you would usually do.

A block of training that involves several weeks of improvement followed by a planned recovery is also known as a mesocycle, and this can last anywhere between two and 12 weeks. When you return from your recovery week you should be refreshed and ready to enter a new mesocycle and make a new set of improvements.

You can introduce a second cycle within your mesocycle, called a microcycle, and this smaller cycle may last only a few days. For example, you might lift heavy on Monday, reduce the weight on Wednesday then go back to lifting heavy on Friday. You would then follow that pattern for a few weeks before changing your exercises.

'Use the same workouts for four to six weeks, but after that you need to take a week off'

Remember the calf

So, if you use realistic load increases and well-timed rest weeks you can keep getting bigger and stronger, right? Not quite. Luckily, for old Milo his cow eventually stopped growing. That's because at some stage the progression has to stop. You can't keep adding 2.5kg to your lifts every week indefinitely. There's only so much your body can do. And progression isn't linear. You'll experience a steep improvement curve to start with and that will slow to incremental changes. It's important to realise that the longer you train the harder it is to make progress.

It may become increasingly challenging to get bigger and stronger once you've been training for years, even if you do use periodisation. But without using periodisation, it's virtually impossible.

At a glance Periodisation

● Structure your periodisation programme according to your goal. If you want strength and hypertrophy, keep your sets and reps the same but increase the weight.

● Don't increase the load you lift each week by more than 2.5 per cent for upper-body moves and five per cent for lower-body exercises.

● Include a rest week at the end of each cycle of weekly load increases. Cycles can last between two and 12 weeks, but four to six is likely to give you the best results.

● You can vary the load you lift within a short amount of time. This is known as a microcycle and increases your chances of adding size and strength.

FREQUENCY

What's the right number of weekly training sessions for the best results? And how much rest do you really need between them?

What many people don't realise is that your muscles don't grow while you're in the gym. Of course, they appear bigger when you're lifting, but that's only because they are filled with blood that creates that 'pumped' look. But while you need weights-based training sessions to make muscles bigger and stronger, it's in the time between your sessions that they actually grow.

This is because while training breaks down the fibres that make up your muscles, it's during the time away from the gym that these damaged cells are repaired. It's this recovery process that adds size and strength. This means that planning your rest is as important as planning your weights sessions, because recovery allows the body to replenish energy stores and repair damaged muscle tissues. So if you are following your training regime to the letter but aren't seeing the gains you'd expect, you may be either resting for too long between

sessions or not resting enough. Taking too long a break between sessions can reduce stimulus momentum, whereas taking too little time to recover can limit your muscle gains while simultaneously increasing your risk of injury and mental boredom.

You'll know when you have had sufficient rest because you'll feel fresh, strong and raring to go. That's because your body has 'super-compensated' from the training so you are stronger. At this point you can push yourself harder than you did before when lifting, and the positive adaptive process repeats itself so you keep getting bigger and stronger.

Easy does it

A rest day doesn't just mean a day away from the gym – though it's vital that it does mean exactly that, otherwise your potential gains will be curtailed – it also needs to be restful. It's no good if your 'recovery' day involves a highly stressful 14-hour day in the office. Remember,

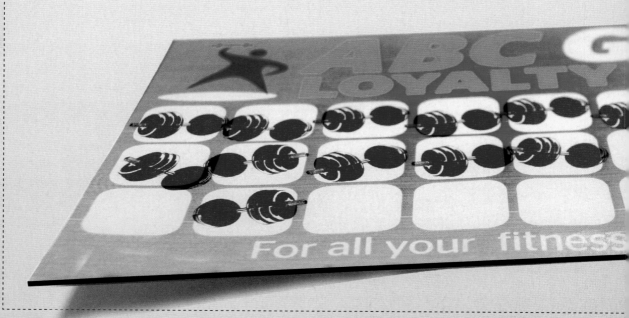

rest is when the magic happens so find some time to relax properly and let your muscles grow.

That said, if fat loss is your primary training aim then it's worth staying active, even on your rest days, by performing some cardio work to keep chipping away at your fat stores.

Own goals

So what's the perfect amount of time needed to recover from a session so that you are in prime condition when you next hit the gym? Again, everything depends on what goals you've set yourself.

If you are training for power then you'll need to leave up to three days between sessions, because power training involves low-rep, high-weight, multi-joint moves, which are very taxing on both the muscles and your central nervous system, so you'll need quality recovery time.

If you want to increase strength, you should aim to train each muscle group

'After lifting, you will grow back stronger if you eat and rest well'

twice a week, which means you should leave between 24 and 48 hours between sessions that target the same muscles. If you are following a split programme, rather than doing total-body sessions (see page 140), it's fine to do upper body one day and legs the next, but you still need to factor in some good-quality rest each week. The same rules apply for building muscle size.

For muscular endurance, which uses lighter weights for a high number of reps, you don't need as much rest because this type of training doesn't do so much fibre damage to the muscle as the others, and so can be performed more frequently. That said, still leave at least 24 hours between sessions, and take one or two rest days a week.

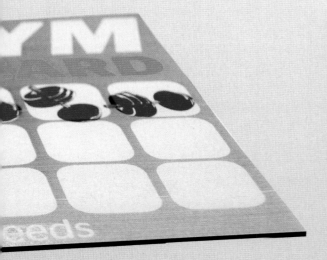

At a glance
Training frequency

- Rest is as important as training in your muscle-building goals because it is during the time between sessions that your muscles are repaired and made bigger and stronger.

- Too little rest means your muscles won't have fully recovered, so you may struggle to lift the same weights for the same sets and reps as before.

- Too much rest between workouts means you are won't be pushing your muscles at the required intensity or giving them sufficient stimulus to grow.

FAILURE

When it comes to building big and strong muscles, failure is the key to success

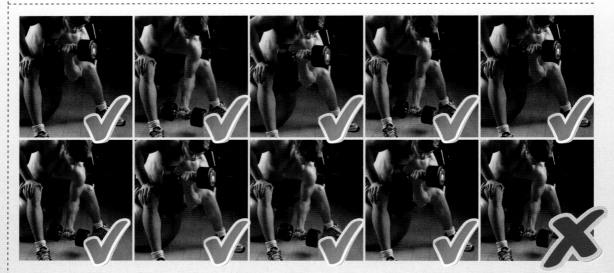

>> Job interviews, your driving test, getting a girl's number. Failure in any of these scenarios is upsetting, frustrating and often downright embarrassing.

But there is one place where failure should be your ultimate objective: the weights room. That's because working your muscles so hard that they fail to complete that final, excruciating rep, is one of the most effective training methods if you want to get stronger, leaner and bigger. If that's your muscle-building ambition, then failure is the only way you can succeed.

In simple terms, training to failure is defined as performing an exercise until you can't do another rep with correct form. So why is this training protocol so good at building muscular size and strength?

When you lift a weight to failure you are overloading your muscles with a level of stress they haven't experienced before. This shocks your body into thinking it is incapable of doing what is required of it so it grows your muscles back stronger. If you don't take your sets to failure and just do three sets of eight comfortable reps instead, then your muscles think that they are already strong enough to perform the task asked of them. The need to grow back stronger isn't so urgent.

Operation overload

When you push your muscles to the absolute limit your brain freaks out and gets your central nervous system to call on as many muscle fibres as it can to start helping out with the lift. Training to failure results in more muscle fibre damage, called microtrauma, because you'll recruit every type of muscle fibre you have available.

This has two significant benefits. First, the more muscle fibres you can recruit and then damage during training, the more fibres grow back bigger and stronger. Second, you are creating a more efficient line of communication between your brain and your muscles, which means that they can react faster and contract with more strength the next time they are called upon – what's known as muscle memory.

Training to failure also places the highest demands on the muscles and the central nervous system, which will have a bigger impact on muscular hypertrophy. Three sets of eight with a sub-maximal load – lifting less than your eight-rep max – does not have the same impact on muscular development or on your neuromuscular, or brain-to-muscle, co-ordination.

The other advantage of training to failure is that you're likely to spend less time lifting.

For strength you will probably only reach failure on your final set, because you'll be aiming for a one- to three-rep max and you will therefore need to do a good number of lighter warm-up sets.

But if you are lifting for size, you need to reach failure between the eighth and 12th rep of each set and only aim for around two sets of a move per muscle group, resting between 90 seconds and four minutes between them. Any more than this is too taxing on your body.

Whether you're lifting for strength or size, you do need to limit number of sets per workout otherwise you run a real danger of burn-out.

Because of the effort involved in lifting to failure stick to no more than three sessions a week, evenly spaced out with between 48 and 72 hours between workouts. This is how long it'll take you to recover sufficiently enough to push a little harder next time.

Failure and fatigue

If you don't leave adequate time between sessions then you are asking for trouble because putting such strain on your central nervous system isn't something you can do regularly. Instead of getting bigger and stronger you'll end up fatigued, with a weakened immune system and all the other nasty side effects of overtraining.

It will also make you weaker because excessive microtrauma of muscle fibres is thought to be counterproductive and might inhibit growth by blunting the anabolic (muscle-building) response you normally get after a hard and successful weights session.

A final consideration is that if you try to train to failure too often you start to lose technique: as soon as correct form goes out the window you are opening the door to an increased chance of injury, especially when you are lifting heavy.

So how do you know what weight you should you be lifting for each exercise? If you are training for strength then you want to lift fewer than six reps per set,

> ## 'When you lift a weight to failure you are overloading your muscles with a level of stress they haven't experienced before'

which would equate to starting with around 80 to 90 per cent of your one-rep max for that move. Whereas, if you want bigger muscles, work with a load that is between 60 and 80 per cent of your one-rep max and aim for between eight and 12 reps per set.

If you are unsure how much weight you should be use when you start your programme of lifting to failure, it's best to start light and take a few sessions to establish your failure point in your target rep range. Remember fewer than six reps per set will build strength, eight to 12 will build size.

If you want to try this protocol there's one final consideration: you have to reach true failure. You'll know when you have because it'll feel like you've been run over and there is just nothing left in your tank. If you are new to training then it's a good idea to have someone more experienced to spot for you, especially during more complicated lifts, to ensure you can complete each set safely.

At a glance Failure

● Training to failure is a strategy in which you're unable to lift the weight with correct form on the final rep of your set.

● This form of overload training shocks your muscles into growing back bigger or stronger.

● Because it is so taxing on your muscles and central nervous system, you need adequate rest between sessions to allow a full recovery.

● Failure to do so will quickly result in overtraining, muscle soreness and even size and strength losses.

TEMPO

The most often neglected training variable – tempo – is one you can't afford to ignore if you want to add serious muscle

>> It's tempting when you first start lifting weights to try and power through your set, banging out the reps as fast as you can so that you can get your workout done and dusted fast.

While this approach can be beneficial if you are an experienced lifter wanting to build explosive power – fast reps train your muscles to contract quickly, resulting in maximum power output – but if you want to build bigger muscles, then you're going to need to spend some time thinking about tempo.

'For strength and conditioning coaches, tempo is another tool – just like sets, reps and weights'

Tempo trap

Tempo is the speed at which you lift and lower the weight during each rep. The longer you take over each rep the harder your muscles must work to manage and control the load. This is commonly known as 'time under tension' (TUT). The longer the TUT, the greater the damage to your muscle fibres, which your body subsequently must repair resulting in bigger and stronger muscles.

Tempo is another tool, just like sets, reps, weight and even exercise selection, that can be tampered with to maximise muscle gains, but most men ignore tempo because they don't recognise or appreciate its importance. You can elicit completely different physiological adaptations by completing the same sets, reps and weight but by varying the tempo.

So what is the right TUT when trying to add muscular size? Research shows that to achieve optimal mass your muscles need to be under tension for between 40 and 70 seconds per set, which means the fastest tempo you should aim for is a two-second up, two-second down approach for sets of ten reps. As you become more experienced you can either stick to this tempo and up the weight, or change the tempo to a two-second up, four-second down approach.

Big returns

To reap the benefits of bigger muscles you may need to leave your ego at the door. It's very tempting to go for the heaviest weights, but it's often more than you can comfortably manage so you are forced to bang out each rep as fast as possible. This results in you using momentum to lift it, rather than placing all the workload on the target muscle group, which is the most efficient way to make them grow.

The answer? Drop the weight. That's the only way to ensure you are hitting the correct tempo on every rep of your set. Although it is important to lift heavy to build muscle, it's better to go a little lighter but extend the length of time under

tension. This will have a far more beneficial effect than going a bit heavier but only for a really short period of time.

Injury free

Performing each rep in a slow and controlled fashion has the additional benefit of preventing injury. Fast and explosive reps shift the stress from the muscles to the connective tissues, such as ligaments and tendons, and this is how injuries often occur in inexperienced lifters who don't know correct form. Resistance training should be focused on high intensity, perfect form and maximum time under tension because this will guarantee muscle growth while minimising your exposure to injury.

Keep it simple

Finally, if you're unsure of how fast or slowly you should be lifting each rep, don't worry. Just ask yourself what your ulitmate training goals are. If you want to train for speed, lift quickly; for maximal strength then lift heavy; for maximal size lift less heavy but more slowly; and for improved endurance capacity then lift lighter for longer. It's that easy.

At a glance Tempo

- Tempo is the speed at which you perform a rep.

- The slower the tempo, the longer your muscles are exposed to the stress of managing the weight. The duration of a rep is called the 'time under tension' (TUT).

- The more damage you can do to your muscles during a session, the bigger and stronger they will grow back.

- Performing each rep very quickly can help build explosive power, but only if you maintain perfect form throughout.

REST

Getting your rest periods right will help you achieve your fitness aims sooner

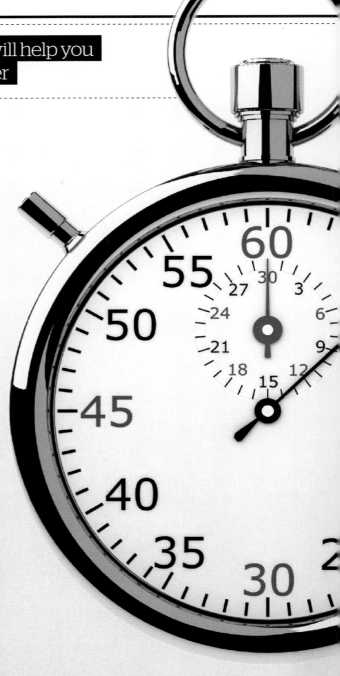

When it comes to building muscle the formula for success is simple. You select a weight, lift it a certain number of times, put it down, rest, then lift again. The 'lifting weights' part is crucial of course, but the period of time that you rest between sets can also have a dramatic impact on the effectiveness of your training session. In fact, rest is a training variable as important as sets, reps, weight and tempo in ensuring you hit your fitness target.

That's because the amount of rest between sets can influence the efficiency, safety and ultimate effectiveness of any given strength-training programme. Why? Because when you lift weights, you do so to push your muscles out of their comfort zone because it's this stress that makes them stronger. But there is only so much work they can do before their energy stores become depleted, hampering their ability to perform additional reps with good form. By resting for a predetermined period you give your body time to resupply the muscle cells with fuel so they can do more lifting.

'How long you rest between sets can have a dramatic impact on your training session'

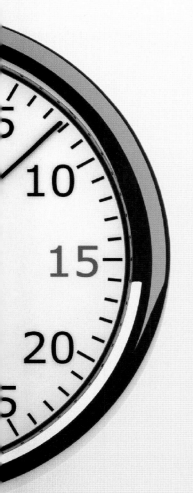

Power play

So how long should you be resting between sets? It depends entirely on your objectives. When training for power, you need to lift moderate to heavy weights at speed, which taxes your central nervous system. This neuromuscular fatigue clogs up the pathways between our brain and muscles, so without sufficient rest you are unable to send the signal that fires up the muscles as quickly as you need to get the bar moving on the next set.

Power training is usually done with complex lifts, such as the snatch and the clean and jerk, and you don't want to attempt potentially dangerous lifts likes these unless everything is firing. You need at least three minutes between sets, if not four or five.

Sizing it up

Hypertrophy or increasing size is all about working the muscles so hard they start to break down, which stimulates your body to repair them so they get bigger. Because you need to work your muscles for between 40 and 70 seconds per set to stimulate growth, this increased time under tension creates a build-up of lactic acid in the muscles, which is painful. Therefore, rest between 60 and 90 seconds between each set, which should be enough time for most of the lactic acid to be removed so you can hit the muscles hard again.

Give me strength

If your aim is to build strength, you need to lift as heavy as you can for around six reps. If you can't stick to this target – either you can't reach six or you reach it too easily – you're using the wrong weight. But while you're finding the right weight, you also need to focus on rest.

When training for gains in strength you need to rest for about the same time as when lifting for power because the volume and intensity is such that it causes both muscular and neuromuscular fatigue. Studies have suggested you can maybe get away with as little as one minute's rest between sets, but three to five minutes is both safer and more effective.

Going the distance

If you want your muscles to be able to handle a load for a longer period of time, you should train with a light weight for high reps and with little time to recover. This trains your muscles to deal with lactic acid build-up more efficiently so you can keep going for longer, so keep rest periods as brief as possible, ideally under 60 seconds.

At a glance Rest

- Rest between sets and exercises lets your muscles replenish their energy stores.

- Not resting for long enough means your muscles won't be as capable of performing the set with good form.

- Resting for too long can result in you not testing your muscles enough to force them to grow back bigger and stronger.

BURN FAT FAST

Torch calories with weights and get the body you've always wanted

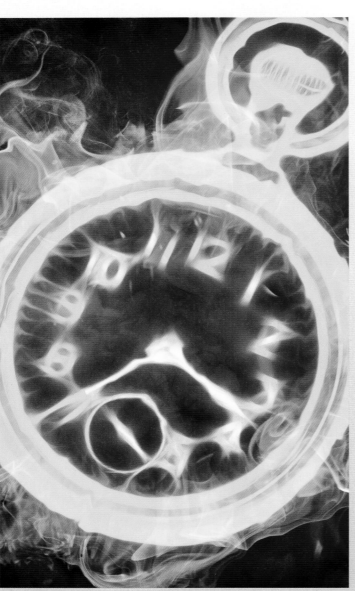

What's the best way to shift that spare tyre around your waist? Long and slow cardio sessions or cutting fat from your diet? The answer is neither. The best approach is lifting weights.

The idea that long but slow cardio sessions – the so-called 'fat-burning zone' – are the best way to lose weight is simply not true. Low-intensity exercise does tap into fat stores for fuel, but it doesn't burn many calories. Training hard and fast, burns calories far more efficiently.

What's more if you perform a lot of cardio then your body can start breaking down muscle tissue to burn as fuel. So, the good news is that your fat-loss training sessions can be a lot shorter. The bad news is that they also need to be a lot harder and be based around lifting weights.

Oxygen debt

Lifting weights is more effective at burning fat than a long, slow run because of the damage it causes to your muscles. A hard weights session creates an oxygen debt in your muscles that must be replenished. This is called excess post-exercise oxygen consumption, or EPOC, and is accompanied by an increased consumption of energy. During this recovery process, fat stores are broken down and free fatty acids are released into the blood where they are used as fuel.

When you lift weights you create small tears in your muscles fibres and these must be repaired. The more muscular damage you create the greater the extent of repair needed, which comes at a higher metabolic cost, so you burn more calories. A steady run will result in higher energy consumption for around 30 minutes after the session, but with weights the effect can last up to 48 hours afterwards, resulting in a far, far greater expenditure of calories.

An additional, longer-term benefit is that weight training will increase your lean muscle mass. Muscle is active tissue that burns calories, which means that if you gain muscle, even at rest your metabolic rate is elevated and your body will be burning more calories. This creates a virtuous cycle where the more muscle you put on, the more fat your body burns.

Get intense
Ready to ditch cardio forever? Not so fast. Lifting weights may burn more calories than slow, steady-state cardio, but high-intensity interval training (HIIT) – a form of short, but intense cardio exercise designed to increase fitness and burn fat – also has a role to play in helping you slim down, especially if you're new to weight training.

The more experienced you are, the more thoroughly you can fatigue your muscles, but if you can't tax your muscles to the extent needed to mobilise fat stores as fuel, then you need to supplement your weight training with some HIIT sessions. Typically, these would involve a warm-up followed by several minutes of all-out effort in cardio exercise – sprinting, cycling or swimming – interspersed with periods of recovery before a cool down.

So what makes intervals the only form of cardio good for torching fat? HIIT also creates an oxygen debt in your muscles that stokes up your metabolism so you continue burning calories long after you've finished training, just as you would if you'd been lifting weights.

When it comes to weight training itself, the best strategy for burning fat is to lift to failure with very short rests between sets because this creates the maximum muscle damage. If you can do three sets of ten reps with ease then you aren't creating an oxygen debt and so won't burn excess calories. Instead do supersets (see page 148) that work different muscle groups so you can work out harder.

In short, to lose fat you need to lift until your muscles literally can't do one more rep before resting for 45 seconds and

'The idea that long but slow cardio sessions are the best way to lose weight is simply not true'

doing another set. Because the rest is so brief, you will have to start dropping the weight you lift after each set, but don't worry about lifting lighter dumb-bells. It may be a blow to your ego in the short-term but you'll get results in the long-term.

Move some metal
Compound moves should form the backbone of your fat-loss session, so stick to squats, lunges, rows, bench and overhead presses, and pull-ups and chin-ups to tax the maximum amount of muscle in the minimum amount of time.

Most compound moves require free weights, such as barbells and dumb-bells, but you shouldn't turn your back on resistance machines.

If your goal is to look better naked then machines may be the better option, if you are new to lifting. Machines take the stability out of each move, allowing you to push harder for greater muscular damage. As you become more advanced start the session with free weights before maxing out on the machines to tax your muscles.

At a glance Burning fat

- Weights are more effective than slow cardio at blitzing fat because your body continues to burn calories long after you've finished training.

- High-intensity interval training is also a good way to burn calories, especially if you are new to lifting weights.

- Keep your rest periods between sets to about 45 seconds for the most effective fat-burning session.

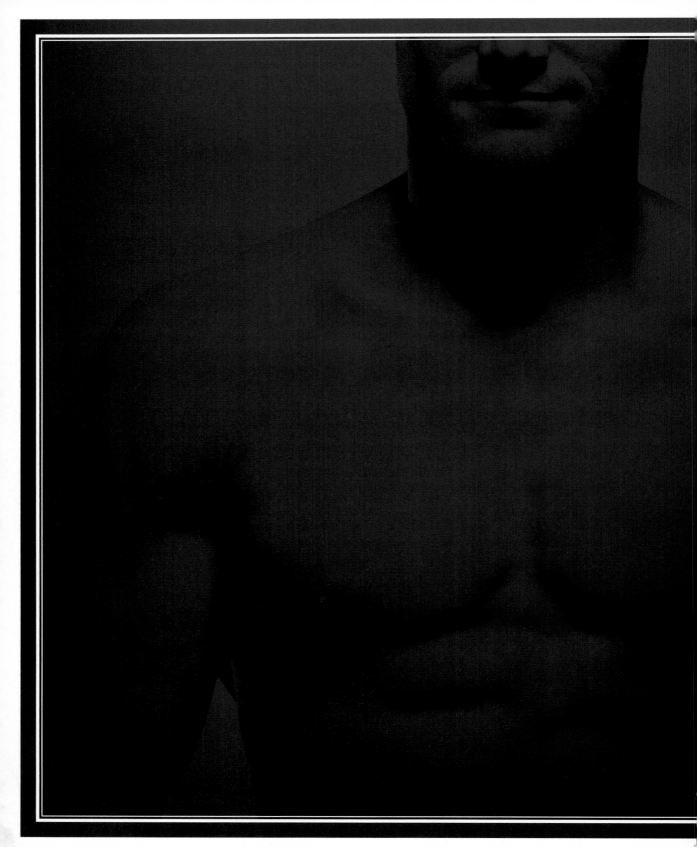

VARY YOUR WORKOUTS

CONTENTS

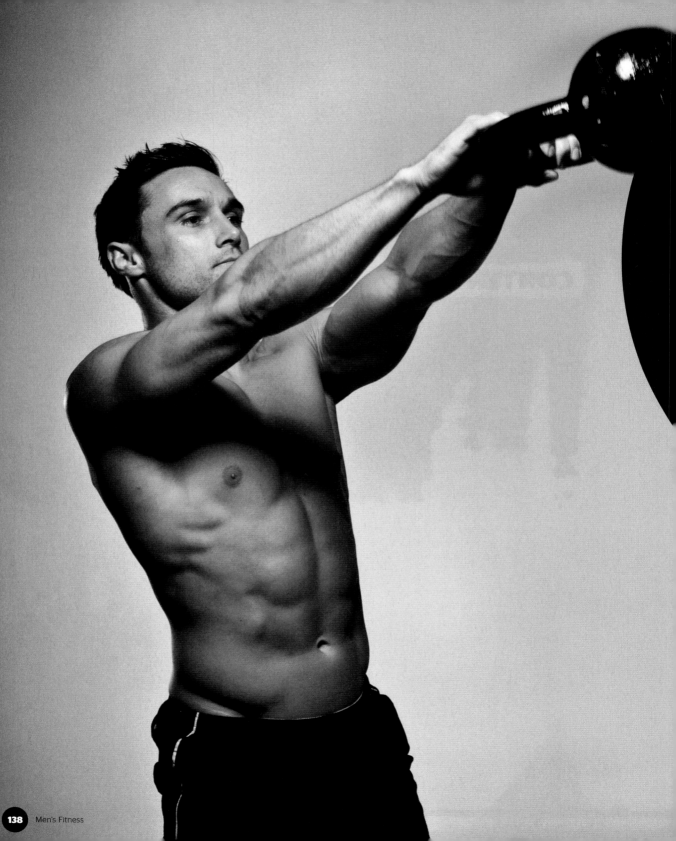

Why vary your workouts?

A change is as good as a rest – and as important – when it comes to building hard muscle

>> Working out is all about change. Of course, the whole point is to change your body, but the best way to achieve this is to regularly change your workouts.

That's not to say that the basic three sets of eight to 12 reps approach doesn't work: it does. But in the same way that you need to regularly change your moves, as discussed in rule four, you also need to perform different workout methods to keep challenging your muscles in new and effective ways.

In this chapter we put some of the most common and popular workout approaches and set strategies under the microscope and, in an easy-to-follow guide, show you what changes you can make to your training programme to ensure your muscles keep growing.

Turn over for a complete guide to the best workout methods and set strategies to add muscle fast.

SPLIT TRAINING

Working different body parts on different days can reap big rewards

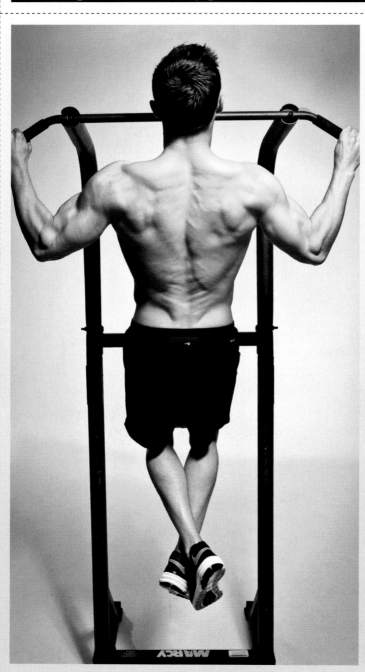

Split – or body part – training involves working specific muscle groups in one session and then focusing on another group of muscles in the next workout. This approach allows you to fully exhaust certain muscles one day, before giving them several days to recover before training them again, during which time you can train other muscle groups.

Each muscle group is typically worked twice a week, with around 48 to 72 hours between these sessions to allow sufficient time for recovery.

Split training is a more advanced approach because it allows you to lift heavy weights on a regular basis, making it one of the best approaches for adding muscle mass quickly and efficiently.

When using this strategy you must increase the weights you are lifting to ensure muscle growth. And while missing the odd session isn't a problem, if you don't stick to the body-part routine you can end up resting for too long between training the same muscle groups, which will stall your progress. Lifting heavy can also result in more muscle soreness, so adequate recovery time is essential for success.

At a glance
Split training

ADVANTAGES

- Great way to add muscle mass.
- Requires just three workouts a week.
- Lets you to focus on hard-to-grow muscle groups.

DISADVANTAGES

- Requires a structured, progressive training programme to be effective.
- Using heavy weights means you may need a spotter.
- Little transfer value to sports because the body doesn't work as a unit.

SPLIT TRAINING SAMPLE WORKOUT

DAY ONE CHEST AND BACK

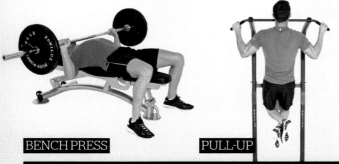

1 Bench press **p60**
2 Incline dumb-bell flye **p85**
3 Incline dumb-bell press **p84**
4 Pull-up **p64**
5 One-arm row **p94**
6 Dumb-bell pullover **p89**

BENCH PRESS

PULL-UP

DAY TWO LEGS

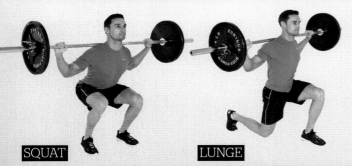

1 Squat **p58**
2 Lunge **p66**
3 Seated hamstring curl **p111**
4 Romanian deadlift **p90**
5 Dumb-bell lateral lunge **p91**
6 Seated calf raise **p111**

SQUAT

LUNGE

DAY THREE REST

DAY FOUR ARMS AND SHOULDERS

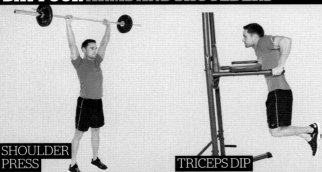

1 Shoulder press **p68**
2 Shrug **p109**
3 Chin-up **p88**
4 EZ-bar biceps curl **p104**
5 Triceps dip **p72**
6 Lying triceps extension **p106**

SHOULDER PRESS

TRICEPS DIP

DAY FIVE REST

DAY SIX REPEAT DAY ONE

TOTAL BODY TRAINING

Working your whole body every session adds muscle and torches fat

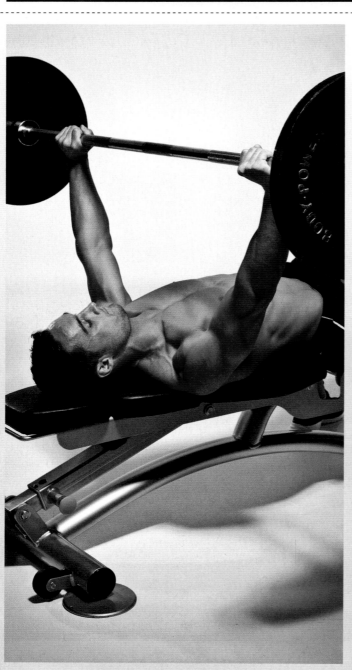

》》 A total body routine involves training every major muscle group each time you hit the gym.

So you'd perform one body-part specific move for a certain number of sets and reps before moving on to another body part.

Alternatively, you could superset antagonistic muscle groups (see page 148) for an even faster and more taxing workout.

This approach promotes muscle gain and burns fat by using compound lifts, which boost the release of testosterone and other growth hormones, but it's also great for working you heart and lungs as you move quickly between exercises that target different muscles and so keep your body guessing what to expect next.

However, it is vital that no muscle groups are neglected during this approach, especially those moves that you don't like. Failure to work the whole body to the same extent can increase your odds of injury and developing muscular imbalances.

At a glance
Total-body training

ADVANTAGES

- Intensive approach that builds muscle and burns fat.

- A session based around compound lifts boosts the release of testosterone and growth hormones.

- Sessions can be performed quickly to minimise time spent training.

- Can provide a good aerobic workout.

DISADVANTAGES

- Working the whole body makes it difficult to fatigue every muscle group.

- Hard to target minor muscle groups.

- Every session can start to feel the same, sapping motivation.

TOTAL BODY SAMPLE WORKOUT

1 DECLINE BENCH PRESS P85
(CHEST AND TRICEPS)

2 BENT-OVER ROW P70
(BACK AND BICEPS)

3 SQUAT P58
(LEGS)

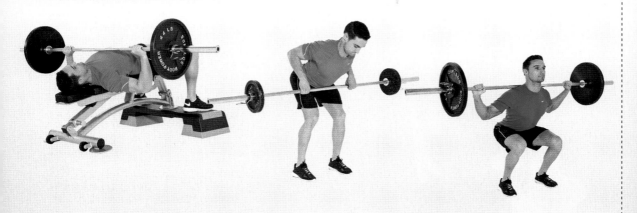

4 GOOD MORNING P86
(LOWER BACK)

5 PUSH PRESS P92
(SHOULDERS)

6 CRUNCH P43
(ABS)

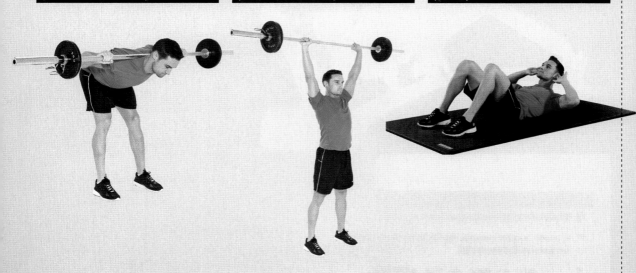

CIRCUIT TRAINING

If you're struggling to find time to squeeze your sessions into an already busy schedule, then circuit training could be the answer

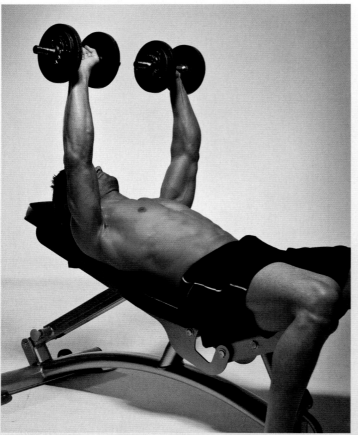

>> If you have a membership with a big gym chain then you've probably seen circuit training classes advertised. Circuit training is a popular type of session because it allows you to work your whole body in a short space of time.

And that's because circuit training is a variety of different moves or stations – anywhere between six and 12 exercises – that are performed back-to-back without rest. Once all of the stations have been completed you then rest for up to three minutes before repeating the circuit again, typically completing three or four full circuits in a single session.

The quick pace and constant switching between exercises and equipment shocks your body and tackles all your major muscle groups, meaning you can get an effective full-body workout in as little as 45 minutes.

Lifting lighter

The intensive nature of this session means that you won't be lifting heavy weights – some stations may only be bodyweight moves – so circuits are better suited for building muscular endurance, burning fat and giving you a decent aerobic workout, than for adding serious muscle mass.

Many gym chains run circuit classes in studios, but you can create your own circuit using resistance machines, free weights or bodyweight moves, or a combination of all three.

At a glance Circuit training

ADVANTAGES

- Works the whole body in a short amount of time
- Provides a good aerobic workout, builds muscular endurance and burns fat.
- Can be done any place, any time, using only bodyweight exercises
- Great transfer value to sports performance.

DISADVANTAGES

- Not ideal for building muscle mass because of the light weights involved.
- Can require a lot of equipment and working in with other people if performed in a gym.
- Need to be motivated to work consistently without stopping for rest.

CIRCUIT TRAINING WORKOUT

1 DUMB-BELL SQUAT P82

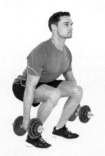

2 DUMB-BELL LATERAL LUNGE P91

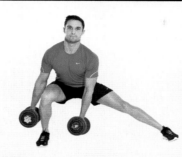

3 CHIN-UP P88

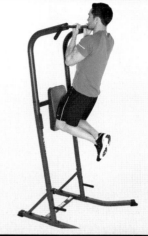

8 MEDICINE BALL PRESS-UP P97

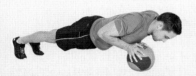

4 TRICEPS DIP P72

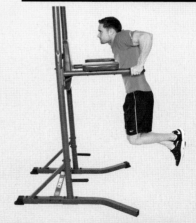

7 SHRUG P109

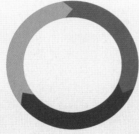

6 DUMB-BELL INCLINE BENCH PRESS P84

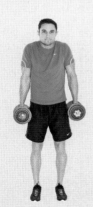

5 DUMB-BELL PULLOVER P89

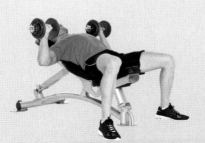
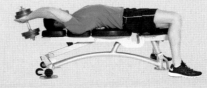

STRAIGHT SETS

The basic – and often the best – way to add lean muscle

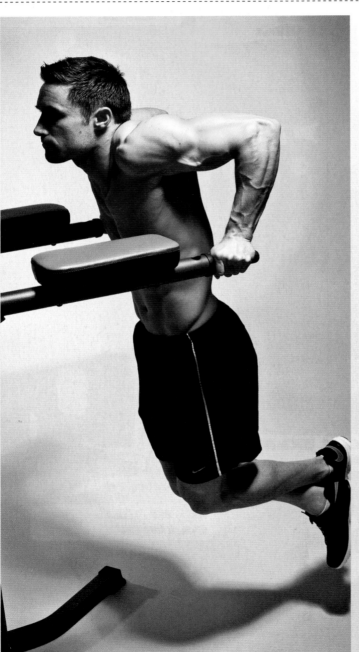

>> Straight sets require you to perform one exercise for a certain number of repetitions – usually eight to 12 – followed by a short rest, then repeating. This is the most basic approach to weightlifting and it can very often be the most effective, especially if you're new to weight training.

STRAIGHT SETS

What?
Performing a certain number of reps of the same exercise, then resting and repeating.

Such as?
In an arms and shoulders session you'd do three sets of ten reps of the shoulder press, then move on and repeat on another exercise.

Why should I do them?
The aim is to work the target muscle group to failure. In this case you would select a weight you can lift ten times for the first two sets, so that by the end of the third set of repetitions your muscles are so fatigued you may struggle to complete all the reps. Straight sets are also great for preparing a muscle group, and its stabilising muscles, for more advanced workouts.

FIT TIP

Getting into the right frame of mind can make a big difference to the effectiveness of your workouts. On your way to the gym, remind yourself of why you started the plan, and imagine how good you'll feel when you reach your goals. If you're having an off-day, and don't feel like training, go anyway, get changed and do a light warm-up. The surge of feel-good hormones may make you change your mind, but don't get discouraged if you do miss a session. Simply pick up where you left off at the next workout.

STRAIGHT SETS SAMPLE WORKOUT

1 SHOULDER PRESS P68

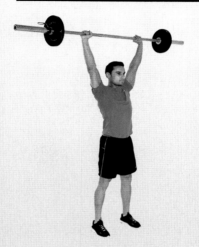

2 SHRUG P109

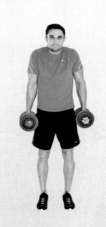

3 CHIN-UP P88

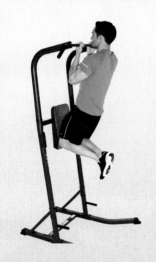

4 ONE-ARM ROW P94

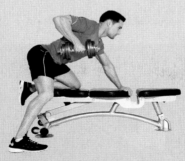

5 LYING TRICEPS EXTENSION P106

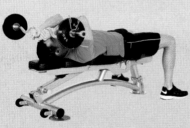
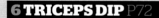

6 TRICEPS DIP P72

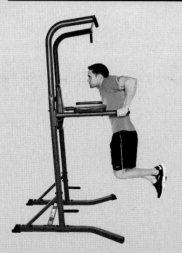

SUPERSETS

Pairing exercises is a fast and effective way to add muscle

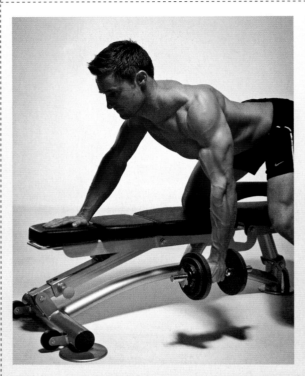

» Supersets are two different exercises done back to back without rest. So, what exactly makes supersets so super? For one thing supersets are a great way to shake up an existing training regime as the increased workload will shock your muscles into growing and, because they allow you to work harder in a far shorter period of time, they improve your muscles' ability to work harder with less rest.

There are a number of different superset workouts you can do. Here are some of the most popular and effective set strategies for adding serious muscle fast.

FIT TIP

To ensure that muscle-growth is even across your body, aim to make your workouts as balanced as possible. This means that you should do as many lower-body moves as upper-body moves; for every pushing motion you perform you should perform a pulling one; and you need to give the same amount of attention to opposing muscle groups, such as biceps and triceps. Also, if one side of your body is stronger than the other, work your weaker side harder to help it catch up.

ANTAGONISTIC SUPERSETS

What?
A superset of two exercises that works opposing muscles groups, affording each group additional recovery time between sets.

Such as?
A set of dumb-bell bench presses (chest and triceps) followed immediately by a set of one-arm rows (back and biceps). Repeat this superset three times.

Why should I do them?
Focusing on different muscle groups provides a more balanced workout in less time and lets you to lift heavier weights in each set, promoting greater muscle gain.

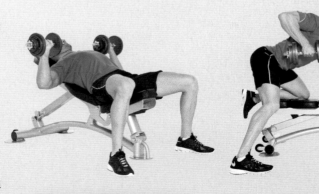

INCLINE DUMB-BELL BENCH PRESS P84

ONE-ARM ROW P94

PERIPHERAL HEART ACTION (PHA) SUPERSETS

What?
A superset of two exercises that work a muscle group in the upper body then one in the lower body without rest in between.

Such as?
A set of lunges (lower body) then bent-over rows (upper body).

Why should I do them?
Alternating between working muscles in opposite ends of your body forces your heart to work really hard to pump blood into the target muscles. This makes the workout more intensive and means you will build muscle and burn fat at the same time.

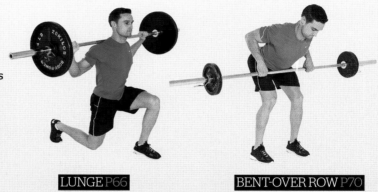

LUNGE P66

BENT-OVER ROW P70

STAGGERED SUPERSETS

What?
These are like straight sets, but you use the rest period between them to work on a hard-to-grow muscle group that requires additional training, such as your calves or core.

Such as?
After a set of good mornings, use your rest period doing seated calf raises to target a muscle groups that requires serious effort to grow bigger.

Why should I do them?
Smaller muscle groups require greater stimulation for growth, and using staggered sets means you can work them even on days when not training them exclusively.

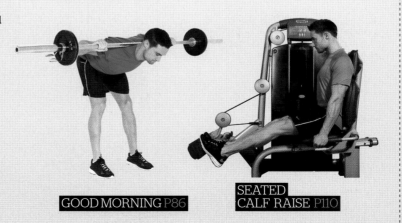

GOOD MORNING P86

SEATED CALF RAISE P110

SUPERSETS

For rapid muscle gains try these advanced superset methods

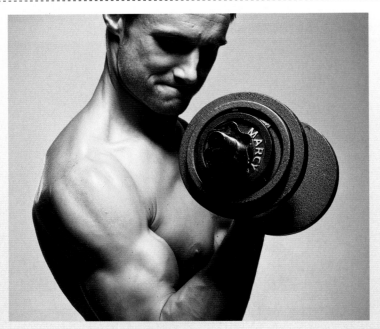

>> These supersets are more advanced workout methods than those on the previous pages, but don't let that put you off. Performed correctly each can be a highly effective way to add lean muscle mass fast, because the intense nature of these supersets recruits the maximum amount of muscle fibres, while also keeping your heart-rate high so your body must eat into its fat stores.

PRE-EXHAUSTION SUPERSETS

What?
Two exercises performed back to back that target the same muscle group. The first move is an isolation exercise, the second is a compound lift.

Such as?
Leg extensions followed by front squats.

Why should I do them?
Fatiguing the muscle with an isolation exercise before exhausting it with a compound move is a highly effective way to break down the most amount of muscle tissue. However, performing a heavy compound lift when tired puts you at a higher risk of injury, so always use a spotter.

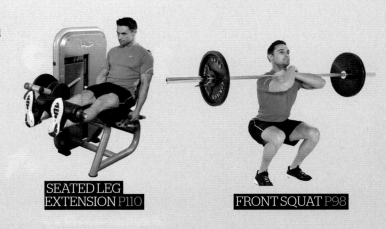

SEATED LEG EXTENSION P110

FRONT SQUAT P98

POST-EXHAUSTION SUPERSET

What?
Two exercises performed back to back that target the same muscle group. The first move is an compound move, the second an isolation exercise.

Such as?
Chins up followed by EZ-bar biceps curls.

Why should I do them?
Performing the compound move first when you are fresh means you can fatigue your muscles, plus the supporting ones, before really blitzing the target muscle with an isolation move. This is a safer strategy than pre-exhaustion but just as effective for building muscle.

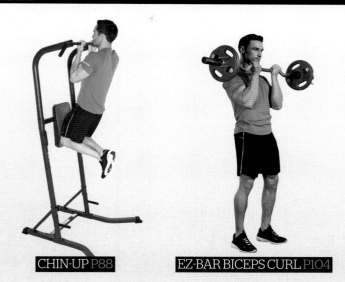

CHIN-UP P88

EZ-BAR BICEPS CURL P104

GERMAN VOLUME TRAINING

What?
A version of an antagonistic superset where you perform two opposing exercises back to back, except you perform ten sets altogether.

Such as?
A set of ten bench presses then ten pull-ups. Rest. Repeat ten times.

Why should I use them?
This approach, made popular by world-renowned strength coach and *Men's Fitness* magazine's muscle expert Charles Poliquin, is designed to pack on the maximum amount of lean muscle in the shortest amount of time. The weight used for each exercise remains the same for every set, and should be around 60 per cent of your one-rep max.

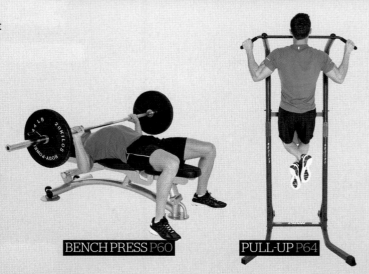

BENCH PRESS P60

PULL-UP P64

TRISETS

Performing three, or even four, moves that target the same muscle group in succession will result in impressive gains

TRISETS

What?
Trisets involve doing three different exercises that target the same muscle group in succession without rest.

Such as?
Ten chin-ups, ten seated cable rows and ten one-arm preacher curls would be a biceps-hitting triset. After the final set you'd rest before repeating.

Why should I do them?
Trisets are great for recruiting additional muscle fibres to help carry out the workload because the muscle fibres you normally rely on become increasingly fatigued as the set progresses. This makes trisets good for building muscular endurance, when using a light weight, and muscular size and strength when using heavier weights.

FIT TIP

Most gyms provide water, but a sensible move is to take a bottle with you so you can sip from it every few minutes to keep your water levels topped up. If you wait until you're thirsty before drinking, the chances are you're already dehydrated and your performance will suffer as a result.

TRI SETS SAMPLE WORKOUT

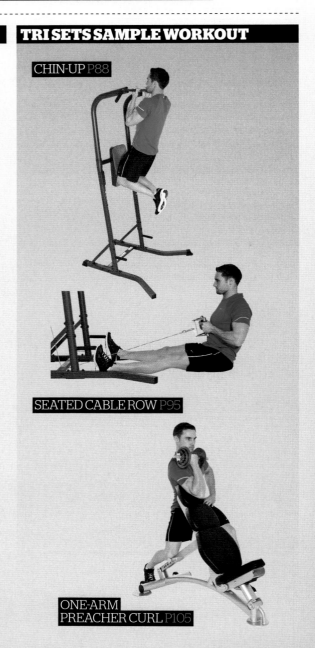

CHIN-UP P88

SEATED CABLE ROW P95

ONE-ARM PREACHER CURL P105

GIANT SETS

What?
A giant set involves four different exercises that target the same muscle group in succession without rest.

Such as?
Triceps dips, close-grip bench press, lying triceps extension, medicine ball press-ups.

Why should I do them?
This is an intense set strategy because the total time your target muscle will be working is significantly longer than with any other type of set. As such, you may need to lower the weights as the set advances – and your muscles become increasingly fatigued – to enable you to perform the desired number of reps. This advanced approach is great for shocking the muscles into growth by really taxing every type of muscle fibre, but you'll need longer to recover after giant set workouts compared to other approaches.

FIT TIP

There are a few rules of gym etiquette that you should follow if you don't want to be ostracised by your fellow members...

● Never hog a machine or a piece of equipment.

● Wipe your sweat off any equipment after you've used it.

● Replace dumb-bells and weight plates on their racks after you've used them.

● Don't trail water from the showers into the changing rooms.

● And don't ogle the girlfriend of the guy in the corner who's bench pressing 200kg.

GIANT SETS SAMPLE WORKOUT

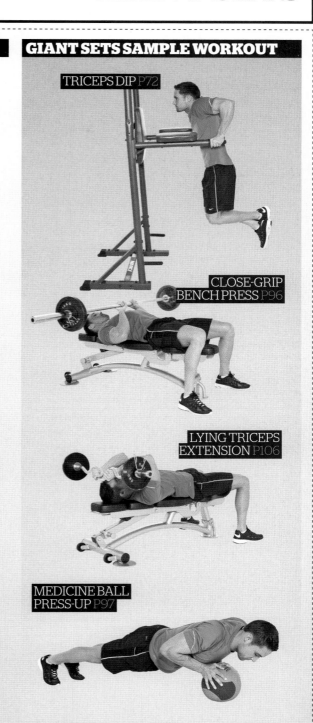

TRICEPS DIP P72

CLOSE-GRIP BENCH PRESS P96

LYING TRICEPS EXTENSION P106

MEDICINE BALL PRESS-UP P97

PYRAMID SETS

Watch muscles grow fast by increasing the weight, while lowering the reps, or working past failure and dropping the weight

PYRAMID SETS

What?
A series of sets of the same exercises in which you increase the weight after each set but reduce the number of reps.

Such as?
To take the deadlift as an example: 15 reps of 60kg, ten reps of 70kg, eight reps of 80kg, four to six reps of 90kg. You can then work back down again.

Why should I do them?
For larger muscle groups pyramid sets are a great way to add mass and strength because your muscles must work harder as the sets progress, which keeps them guessing and puts them out of the comfort zone, resulting in bigger gains.

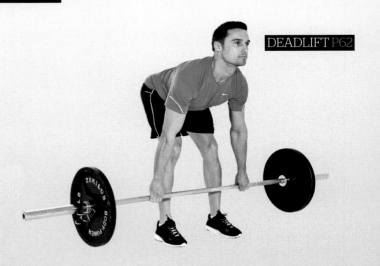

DEADLIFT P62

FIT TIP

Proper form is critical in pyramid sets to avoid injury, especially as the weight increases. Make sure you are comfortable with each phase of a move and how they come together for each rep before attempting heavy lifts.

PYRAMID SETS CHART

At the end of each set increase the weight but reduce the number of reps

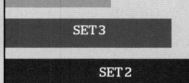

WEIGHT

SET 4
SET 3
SET 2
SET 1

REPS

DROP SETS

DROP SETS

What?
A series of sets of the same exercise in which you start with a heavy weight and lift that until fatigued, then reduce the weight and do a new set to fatigue, pausing to rest between sets.

Such as?
Starting a incline dumb-bell flyes with 20kg dumb-bells, working to failure, then immediately grabbing the 15kg weights and continuing like this until you can't do a single rep, even with a really light dumb-bell.

Why should I do them?
To work the target muscle to complete fatigue and damage as many muscle fibres as possible so that they grow back bigger. Keep the weight drops small between sets and your final set should be with a weight about 20 per cent of the start weight. These sets really tax the muscles, so leave a good few days between sessions to allow for sufficient recovery.

INCLINE DUMB-BELL FLYE P85

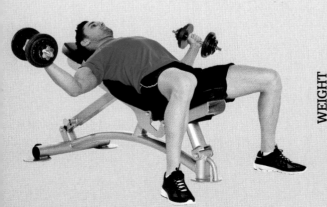

FIT TIP

One of the keys to making progress is to record your progress. If you don't know what you lifted last session and for how many sets and reps, you won't know what to aim for next time, or know whether you are making regular improvements. A written record is evidence of your progress and helps you to stick to your training programme.

DROP SETS CHART

At the end of each set, lower the weight and continue lifting until you reach failure again. Then lower the weight and continue.

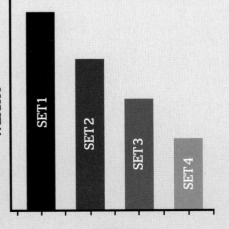

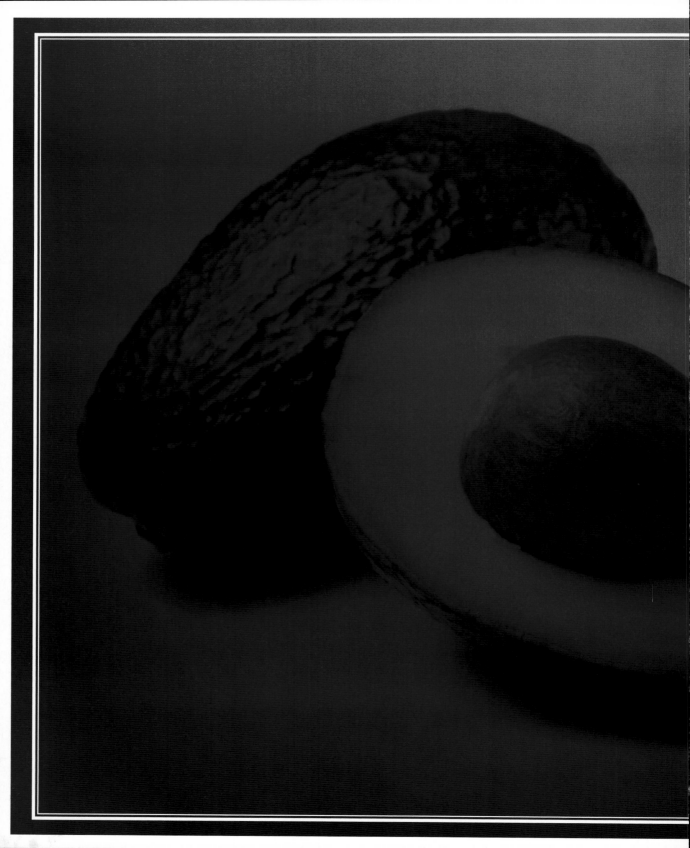

EAT TO BUILD MUSCLE

CONTENTS

EAT FOR A BETTER BODY

Good nutrition is half the battle to gaining muscle, so follow these basic rules and start seeing a real change to your body

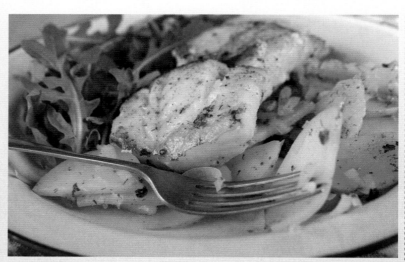

1 Watch your calories

If you eat fewer calories each day than you burn off through activity you'll lose weight; eat more, and you'll gain weight. Of course, whether you gain that weight as fat or muscle will depend on the kind of foods you eat and the training you do.

2 Get the balance right

Nearly all your calories come from a combination of the three main macronutrients: carbohydrates, protein and fats.

Carbohydrates are vital to provide the muscle glycogen that fuels your workouts and should make up about 50-60 per cent of your total calorie intake.

Protein is needed to grow new tissue in your body and is therefore of interest to anyone building muscle. The optimum intake of protein for muscle-gainers is between 1.5g and 2g of protein per kilo of bodyweight, but, depending on your body type (see page 16), it doesn't hurt to take in a bit more to ensure that you are hitting your daily protein targets.

Fat is a nutrient that many people try to avoid altogether, but it can help you absorb vitamins, improve athletic performance and protect joints and tendons against injury. However, fat is a very energy-dense nutrient, containing nine calories per gram compared to around four calories for carbs and protein, so you only need about 50-60g of fat a day.

3 Eat the right stuff

The simplest rule when deciding what to eat is: keep it natural. Processed foods – biscuits, cakes, ready meals, fizzy drinks, crisps – tend to be high on calories but low on essential nutrients, so they're poor at fuelling workouts and rebuilding muscle but good at making you fat.

Carbohydrates provide the energy you need to train hard, but they can also be responsible for altering your blood-sugar levels and making you store fat, so the simplest rule to follow is to make the majority of your carbs unrefined, unprocessed, low on the glycaemic index and high in fibre. This includes vegetables, wholegrain bread, wholewheat pasta, oats and beans, which release energy slowly, ensuring you'll always have enough stored glycogen in your muscles for a workout.

Protein-rich foods include lean meat, fish, eggs and dairy produce. Lower-quality protein can also be found in nuts, seeds and beans. Aim to eat a wide variety of protein-rich foods to get the full range of muscle-building amino acids.

Fats aren't all bad. The ones to avoid are trans fats, which means skipping cakes, biscuits and margarine and cutting back on red meats and cheese. The fats you need are monounsaturates and polyunsaturates, found in olive oil, nuts, seeds and oily fish. These include omega 3 and omega 6 fatty acids, which have been proven to aid strength and aerobic training and protect the body from injuries.

4 Eat at the right times

When you're training hard you want to eat about an hour or two before your workouts and again immediately afterwards. Your snacks should include both carbs and protein to help restore glycogen levels in your muscles and repair muscle tissue. A post-workout snack might be a bagel with salmon and cream cheese, or a tuna and pasta salad.

For the rest of the day, eat small meals at regular intervals of two or three hours, with the aim of having some protein with every meal. This way you keep your glycogen levels topped up and prevent your body from breaking down and using the proteins that you need for muscle building.

5 Take on fluids – but not booze

When you work out you sweat a lot, and you need to need to replace that fluid with water. The trick is to ensure that you hydrate yourself before you get thirsty, not afterwards.

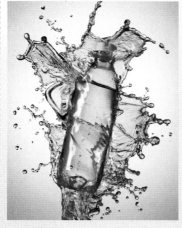

Dehydration will impact on your performance in the gym and can affect the way your body stores fat and repairs muscle owing to poor organ function. Take a water bottle with you to the gym and sip from it every few minutes. Over the course of a day you should aim to take in about two to three litres of water in total.

Alcohol, on the other hand, you can do without. It can have a catabolic effect on your muscles, meaning it prevents them from developing properly. If you are serious about gaining muscle mass, keep pub sessions to a minimum.

6 Supplements are useful, but don't rely on them

Sports supplements, such as protein powders and energy drinks, shouldn't be seen as an alternative to a good diet. Eating healthily

'Processed foods like biscuits, cakes and ready meals are poor at rebuilding muscle but good at making you fat'

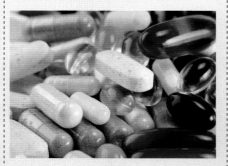

is more important than glugging down shakes, but they do have one advantage: convenience.

It can be tough to consume all the calories you need every day through food alone, and it's much easier to take a protein shake to the gym than to whip up a chicken salad, so supplements can be useful for anyone serious about gaining muscle and losing fat. Also, people who do a lot of exercise can need extra vitamins C and E, so a supplement of these can be handy if you struggle to get enough in your diet.

If you do use supplements, be sure to pick a reputable brand and follow the guidelines on the packaging. See page 170 for our complete guide to supplements.

THE NEW RULES OF FOOD

Eating properly shouldn't take a diploma, so we've simplified everything you need to know into seven simple rules

What you eat is every bit as important to your fitness as what you do in the gym, but every week different fad diets and scare stories hit the news, making it impossible to work out which bits of advice to follow. It's easy to justify bad choices – after all, scientists and nutritionists are constantly changing their minds, right? Wrong. Those in the know agree on what you should be putting in your mouth – and what's more, it's much simpler than you'd expect. Here, we've distilled that collective wisdom into seven rules. Write them down on a postcard, stick it on your fridge – and tuck in.

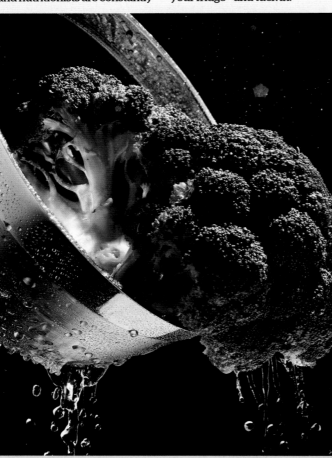

RULE ONE
GREEN IS GOOD

We're starting with this because it could define how you think about the rest of your diet: there's no such thing as too much veg, especially if you're talking about vegetables grown above ground. Regardless of what else you're eating, your plate should be about half-full of them.

The Food Standards Agency (FSA) has introduced the 'eatwell plate' to replace the traditional food pyramid as the government-endorsed illustration of what to eat. This suggests that roughly a third of your diet should come from fruit and veg. But it also suggests that another third should be made up of bread, rice and other starchy foods.

This is not the way to a hard, lean body, because the fundamental problem with starchy carbohydrates is that they cause sudden and prolonged rises in blood sugar, which can provoke a slew of biochemical imbalances that predispose you to weight gain, type 2 diabetes and other diseases.

Besides, there's nothing in them that you can't get elsewhere. If you're going to eat carbohydrate, make sure it's more nutritious carbohydrate with slower sugar release, which is almost every vegetable apart from the potato. It's also a bit of an oversimplification to put fruit and vegetables together, as the FSA plate does. Yes, they're both good for you, but they're radically different nutritionally. If you're getting your five a day from fruit alone, then your blood sugar levels will be going crazy throughout the day from the high fructose content.

If you want to get lean to show off your abs then remember: you'd have to eat half a kilo of asparagus to ingest the same number of carbs as in a single wholemeal pitta bread.

BITE-SIZED SUMMARY
Make vegetables the foundation of your diet, along with two pieces of fruit a day. Vary them as much as you can.

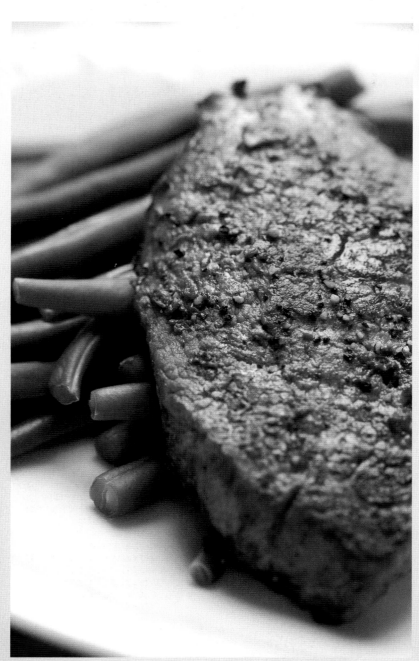

RULE TWO
EAT PROTEIN WITH EVERYTHING

Sooner or later, you'll run into someone at the gym, office or all-you-can-eat buffet who raises an eyebrow at the amount of protein you're eating. Some may even tell you that it can be bad for your health.

The truth is the only studies that have ever suggested that protein can cause kidney problems were done on people who had pre-existing kidney problems. The studies showing that it's harmful to anyone else simply don't exist.

Protein is one of the most important components of the diet and when you eat a high-protein diet, you're generally less hungry, eat less and lose weight as a result.

So what's the right amount? Estimates vary from one to four grams per kilo of bodyweight, per day, but most nutritionists agree on two grams as the minimum. As for how much you can digest at one sitting, a 2009 study from Canada's McMaster University found that increasing protein intake per meal only increased protein synthesis (raised the amount the body could use) up to a dose of roughly 20g – though the study focused specifically on egg proteins. Stick to a two-to-one ratio of vegetables to protein in every meal, by sight.

BITE-SIZED SUMMARY

It's virtually impossible to eat too much protein, although you could easily be not getting enough. Make sure you make it a part of every meal.

THE NEW RULES OF FOOD

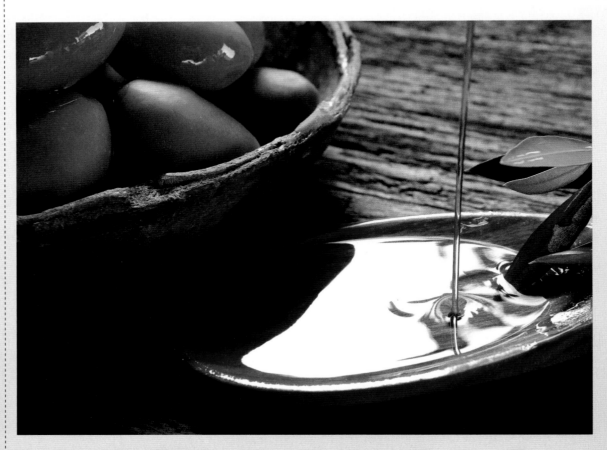

RULE THREE
DON'T FEAR FAT

Although most of us know that eating some fat is essential to a healthy diet, it's all too easy to make a mental connection between eating fat and getting fat, so you end up simply skipping it. Trouble is, that usually means eating something that's worse for you.

One possible issue the FSA has with fat is that it's more calorific, per gram, than carbohydrate or protein, but if you're worried about your weight one of the keys is to eat foods that are genuinely satisfying because you'll eat less of them, which you'll often do with fat. You also want to avoid spikes in insulin, which is what you're going to get if you're eating carbs instead.

There's also the issue of whether it's OK to eat saturated fat – typically demonised as a cause of high cholesterol. Thinking is shifting towards the positive. Some recent studies have failed to find any link between saturated fats and heart disease.

Hydrogenated and trans fats are a different story, with the research sounding alarm bells, but when you look at naturally occurring fats such as the ones in red meat, avocado and nuts, there seems to be no cause for concern.

After all, humans have evolved to eat saturated fats, so it seems strange that it's only in the past 50 years that have they become bad for us. Whereas grains, a relatively recent addition to our diets in evolutionary terms, may not be so easily processed by our bodies.

BITE-SIZED SUMMARY
Avoided partially hydrogenated fats – especially trans fats. Don't worry too much about the rest.

RULE FOUR
START AS YOU MEAN TO GO ON

You always eat breakfast, of course, because you know it's the most important meal of the day and that skipping it slows your metabolism to a crawl. But are you still getting it wrong? You will be if you listen to the FSA's recommendation that you 'base your breakfast on bread or breakfast cereals', and 'wash it down with some fruit juice'.

Eating a high-carb breakfast will give you low blood sugar by mid morning, making you more likely to snack on more high-carb foods, which creates a vicious circle of snacking.

So instead of starting your day on toast or cereal, have something low-carb that's more nutritionally sustainable such as oats with berries and nuts or scrambled eggs with smoked salmon.

Alternatively, just see off whatever's in the kitchen because last night's leftovers are one of the best (and cheapest) things you can eat, assuming you're eating right in the first place.

BITE-SIZED SUMMARY

Think of breakfast like any other meal: you need a blend of protein, fats and fruit or veg.

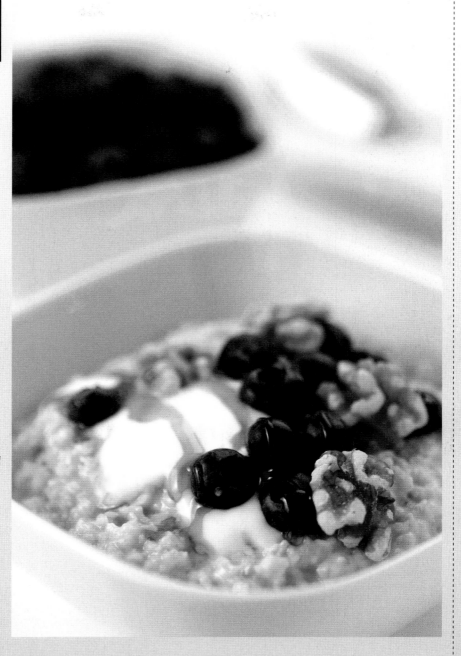

THE NEW RULES OF FOOD

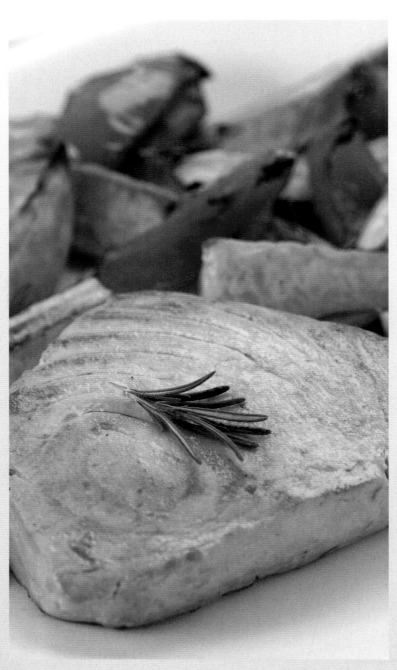

RULE FIVE
ALL CALORIES ARE NOT EQUAL

Calories: the government wants restaurants to include them on menus and women frantically add them up in the Tesco Express snack aisle, but should we really award them so much importance when it comes to fat loss?

No, because calories are not a good indication of what a food is like and the effect it's going to have on your metabolic rate. Would you really say that a couple of poached eggs are 'the same' as a can of Coke, just because they contain a similar number of calories? Of course not.

Also, counting calories makes it too easy to justify bad dietary decisions. Ever heard a friend say that they can eat what they want because they'll burn it off at the gym? They couldn't be more wrong. In fact, the more active you are, the better your nutrition needs to be.

Far more important than calorie content is your food's glycaemic load (GL), which indicates how much of a blood sugar spike it'll give you – yet no one's asking food manufacturers to list glycaemic load on their packaging.

But, if you've stuck with us so far that shouldn't be a problem. Steering clear of starchy food and sugar means you're already avoiding foods with high GL.

You can also slow the absorption rate of high-GL foods, and so help prevent blood-sugar wobbles, by eating them with more protein-heavy foods like chicken or tuna.

BITE-SIZED SUMMARY
Think quality, not quantity. Eating nutritious food is far, far better than sticking rigidly to a 2,000-calorie-a-day limit especially if those calories come from ready meals, pizzas, beer and crisps.

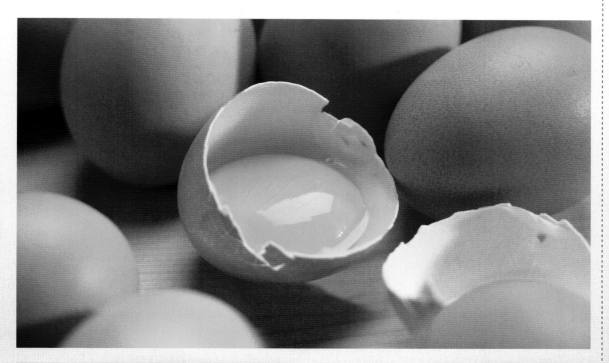

RULE SIX
FREE RANGE IS KEY

Just in case that bulk-value crate of cage-raised eggs is starting to look tempting, let us point out that organic and free-range meat and fish is better for you.

Free range chickens, for example, have a more varied diet and they get a lot more exercise than their battery cousins. And this allows the development of more muscle, which tends to contain more zinc, vitamins B, A and K, amino acids, iron, selenium and phosphorus.

Also, farm-raised salmon have been found to contain up to eight times the level of carcinogens as wild fish, thanks to their cramped conditions and poor-quality feed, while grass-fed beef tends to have much higher levels of conjugated linoleic acid and omega 3s than the kind fed on grain. Think of it this way and free-range feels less like a frivolous luxury. In fact it's so nutritionally dissimilar to cage-reared it's basically a different food.

BITE-SIZED SUMMARY
Eat free-range chickens, grass-fed beef and wild-caught salmon when you can. If you don't know where it's from, chances are the answer's not going to be good.

RULE SEVEN
EAT REAL FOOD

Follow this rule, and you'll end up following all the other rules almost by default.

As a simple rule of thumb eat only food that grows out of the ground or once had a face. Or alternatively, simply think like your hunter-gatherer ancestors or at least back to a pre-industrialised world . When you're looking at something on the shelf, ask yourself if it would have existed 5,000 years ago. If the answer's no, it probably isn't something that you should be eating.

You may find it easier to stick to the outer aisles of the supermarket, which is where all the fresh produce is usually kept for ease of transportation, and away from the interior where everything's canned, processed or packed full of preservatives. Avoid things containing preservatives that you can't spell or ingredients you wouldn't keep in the kitchen. Eat things that will rot eventually, so that you know they're fresh. And try to enjoy it.

BITE-SIZED SUMMARY
Eat food, not products pretending to be food.

MUSCLE MEAL PLAN

Eat like a caveman to add power and prevent weight gain

>> For millions of years humans had no refined sugars or processed foods. So although such modern grub may be tasty and convenient, your body hasn't evolved to deal with it very well – and it usually encourages fat storage. This meal plan, created by nutritionist Christine Bailey (advancenutrition.co.uk) and based on the *Paleo Diet for Athletes,* replaces processed sugary foods and carbs with fresh fruit, nuts, seeds and animal proteins – the staple Stone Age foods. It has plenty of healthy unsaturated fats and branched-chain amino acids, which as well as aiding fat loss will help muscle development and anabolic function. If you're still peckish in the day grab a handful of nuts or drink a low-carb, high-protein shake.

42 prehistoric meals to keep the flab at bay

MONDAY	TUESDAY	WEDNESDAY

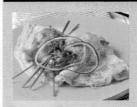

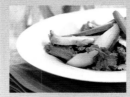

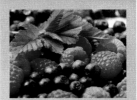

MONDAY

Breakfast
1 grapefruit. 2-egg omelette with ½ an avocado, spinach and 2 chopped tomatoes.

Snack
1 banana.

Lunch
150g grilled cod fillet with lemon juice and freshly ground black pepper. Green salad with lemon juice and 1tsp olive oil, 50g sugar snap peas, cucumber slices, ½ a red pepper and 2tbsp black olives. Bowl of blueberries and diced melon.

Snack
3 cold lean beef slices. Carrot sticks.

Dinner
Ginger baked turkey. 100g fresh raspberries with 2tbsp flaked almonds.

Snack
30g macadamia nuts. Handful of raisins.

DAILY TOTAL
1,840 calories, 163g carbs, 130g protein, 79g fat

TUESDAY

Breakfast
150g sautéed prawns with 6 sliced mushrooms and ½ chopped red pepper. 150g fresh pineapple slices.

Snack
Smoked salmon slices. Carrot and celery sticks.

Lunch
Chicken and avocado salad. 1 apple. 30g almonds.

Snack
1 hard-boiled egg. 2 oatcakes.

Dinner
300ml home-made vegetable soup. Pan-fried venison with cherry sauce.

Snack
2 satsumas.

DAILY TOTAL
1,713 calories, 147g carbs, 156g protein, 60g fat

WEDNESDAY

Breakfast
Bowl of blueberries and raspberries. 2 poached eggs with asparagus and 4 grilled mushrooms.

Snack
Handful of seeds. 1 apple.

Lunch
300ml home-made vegetable soup. Cold venison steak served with a bag of mixed salad leaves, ½ red pepper, 2tbsp black olives, sliced cucumber, celery and 1 tomato. Slices of melon.

Snack
2 slices of ham. Carrot sticks.

Dinner
Chicken and cashew nut stir-fry. Sliced fresh pineapple.

Snack
1 banana. Handful of macadamia nuts.

DAILY TOTAL
1,956 calories, 179g carbs, 130g protein, 87g fat

THURSDAY

Breakfast
Slices of melon with brazil nuts. 3 slices of lean roast beef with 2 baked tomatoes.

Snack
1 apple. Handful of raisins and almonds.

Lunch
300ml home-made vegetable soup. Grilled pork fillet with spinach salad (handful of baby spinach leaves, mixed lettuce leaves, ½ red onion, ½ red pepper, chopped fresh cucumber slices, celery). 1 satsuma.

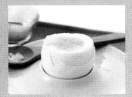

Snack
1 hard-boiled egg. Carrot sticks.

Dinner
Baked butternut squash and turkey casserole.

Snack
2 oatcakes. Smoked salmon slices.

DAILY TOTAL
1,841 calories, 201g carbs, 138g protein, 60g fat

FRIDAY

Breakfast
Bowl of cherries. 2 scrambled eggs with 5 asparagus spears.

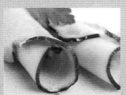

Snack
2 slices of ham, sliced cucumber and celery.

Lunch
Leftover squash and turkey casserole. Large mixed salad.

Snack
Handful of raisins and almonds. 1 pear.

Dinner
300ml home-made vegetable soup. Baked salmon fillet with lemon juice (cook an extra salmon fillet for Saturday) served with 60g steamed carrots, 60g sugar snap peas, 60g green beans and 1 baked sweet potato.

Snack
1 banana. Handful of cashew nuts.

DAILY TOTAL
1,816 calories, 185g carbs, 120g protein, 71g fat

SATURDAY

Breakfast
Bowl of blueberries and raspberries. 1 cold salmon fillet with pan-fried tomatoes and mushrooms.

Snack
4 oatcakes with ham.

Lunch
Grilled turkey breast with 1 baked sweet potato, salad leaves, cucumber, sugar snap peas, ½ a red pepper, 2tbsp black olives and ½ a red onion. Slices of fresh pineapple.

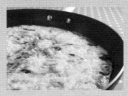

Snack
100g cooked prawns. Celery and carrot sticks.

Dinner
Frittata with 2 eggs, 3 new potatoes, spinach leaves, 1 red pepper. Steamed broccoli and carrots and salad.

Snack
1 banana. Handful of macadamia nuts.

DAILY TOTAL
1,827 calories, 172g carbs, 133g protein, 72g fat

SUNDAY

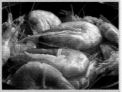

Breakfast
100g cooked prawns with green beans. 1 chopped apple and 2tbsp seeds.

Snack
2 slices of ham and 2 tomatoes.

Lunch
Lemon crab salad. Slices of melon.

Snack
2 oatcakes. Smoked salmon slices.

Dinner
Pork stir fry. 1 satsuma.

Snack
2 oatcakes. Handful of almonds and raisins

DAILY TOTAL
1,746 calories, 159g carbs, 140g protein, 66g fat

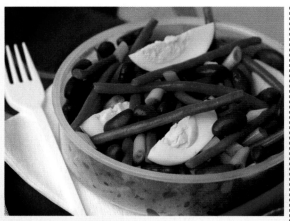

Two-bean muscle salad

You don't need meat for a protein-packed post-workout snack

>> Although lean meat and fish are great sources of protein there are plenty of vegetarian options. This salad is easy to make and provides your body with a good dose of protein to help you build muscle and recover faster after a hard workout.

What you will need

200g green beans
420g can red kidney beans, drained and rinsed
2 hard-boiled eggs, quartered
3 spring onions, chopped

What you will get

Kidney beans
A virtually fat-free source of high-quality, muscle-building protein. Kidney beans are also rich in fibre, which keeps you feeling full for longer and is crucial for digestive health.

Green beans
One portion of green beans provides 25 per cent of your daily vitamin K requirement, which helps to build strong bones. They're also a great source of both magnesium and potassium, which work together to help lower blood pressure.

Eggs
Eggs contain all the crucial amino acids that your muscles need to build and repair themselves. They're also packed with testosterone-boosting zinc, which is crucial to help you build muscle and burn fat.

Spring onions
The quercetin and vitamin C found in spring onions work in synergy to kill harmful bacteria and boost your immune system, while their high levels of chromium can help to keep blood sugar levels in check.

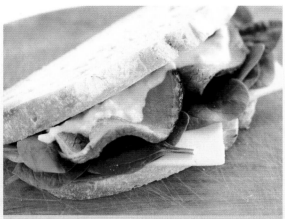

Beef for bulk

Fuel your training with this tasty, meaty sandwich

>> Eat this fitness-boosting snack an hour or so before your workout. Its quality carbs will give you the energy to get through a tough session, while the protein and creatine will help you build muscle.

What you will need

It's insulin release is even lower than that caused by wholemeal bread.

2 slices of sourdough bread
2 thick slices of beef
2 thin slices of cheddar
Handful of spinach
1tsp of horseradish

What you will get

Cheese
An excellent source of casein, which is a high-quality muscle-building protein. The vitamin D in the beef also helps your body to absorb bone-strengthening calcium from the cheese.

Sourdough bread
Sourdough is low on the glycaemic index (GI), so releases its energy slowly.

Beef
Beef contains high levels of slow-digesting protein – essential for muscle growth – and creatine, which increases muscle size by drawing water into your muscle cells.

Spinach
These green leaves are full of iron, which supplies working muscles with oxygen. It also contains betacarotene, an antioxidant that will soothe post-training stiffness and pains.

Horseradish
Horseradish contains high levels of potassium, which helps your muscles and nerves to function properly and lowers your risk of high blood pressure.

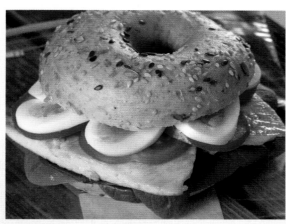

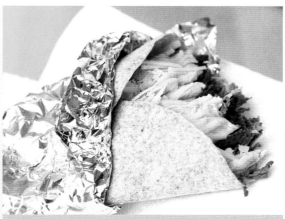

Energy bagel

This snack will fuel your training and help you build serious muscle

>> Snack on this bagel before training and the carbs will help to keep your glycogen levels topped up, ensuring your body uses them for fuel, rather than your protein stores. It will also help to energise your workouts.

 ### What you will need

1 wholemeal bagel
2 thick slices of turkey
1 hard-boiled egg, sliced
1 sliced tomato
Handful of spinach

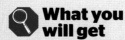 ### What you will get

Wholemeal bagel
A wholemeal bagel is packed with high-quality carbs for a sustained energy boost. It also helps contribute towards your daily requirement of dietary fibre.

Turkey
Turkey is a lean and low-calorie way to pack on muscle, thanks to its generous protein content. It is also rich in selenium, which strengthens the immune system and wards off the free-radical damage caused by exercise.

Egg
Eggs contain all the essential amino acids that your muscles need to build and repair themselves. They are also packed with testosterone-boosting zinc, which helps you to build muscle and burn fat.

Tomato
Vitamin C makes a hefty contribution to your amino acid metabolism, which helps the body to form new muscle. Tomatoes contain betacarotene and lycopene, which reduce inflammation and muscle soreness.

Spinach
Spinach is full of iron, which supplies working muscles with oxygen. Its high vitamin K content will also strengthen your bones.

Recovery wrap

Building post-workout muscle has never been easier or tastier

>> Chicken and cheese wraps are a fast-food restaurant staple, but use your own fresh ingredients and they turn into superb muscle-building snacks. Blending quality carbs, protein and fats with a variety of essential vitamins, this grilled chicken wrap will help you to pack on bulk and recover faster after a testing workout.

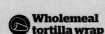 ### What you will need

1 wholemeal tortilla wrap
80g grilled chicken breast, shredded
20g cheddar cheese, grated
30g cabbage, shredded

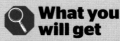 ### What you will get

 Grilled chicken breast
As well as providing a large dose of lean protein vital for muscle growth and recovery, chicken also contains plenty of vitamin B3, which will help to prevent fat storage.

Wholemeal tortilla wrap
A wholemeal tortilla wrap is packed full of carbs to help replenish your muscles, and it's also full of energy-boosting B vitamins.

Cheddar cheese
This dairy product is a great source of casein, a high-quality muscle-protecting protein. It also contains high levels of bone-strengthening calcium.

Cabbage
Cabbage is high in immune system-boosting vitamin C as well as plenty of dietary fibre, which your body needs to maintain a healthy digestive system.

SUPPLEMENTS

Supplements promise everything from torching your love-handles to sculpting your pecs – but do they work? And which ones do you really need? Our comprehensive guide explains all you need to know

>> Whether you regularly pack a protein shake in your gym bag or just chug the occasional isotonic sports drink, chances are you've used supplements at one time or another. Trouble is, the whole process can get a bit confusing – with every supplier claiming that its brand is better filtered, or more efficient, or will pack on more muscle – to the point where you feel like you need a degree in chemistry just to understand what you're putting into your body.

Don't worry – help is at hand. The science may be baffling, but we've put together the definitive guide that details all the latest developments in supplement science: what you need, when you need it, why you need it, and what – if any – are the potential pitfalls.

It's possible you'll find something that will send your training gains through the roof – or you might just learn a bit more about the stuff you're already using. Either way, next time you put in a hard day at the gym, you'll know that you're getting the nutritional backup you need.

PROTEIN

What is it?
Protein is part of the structure of every cell and tissue in your body, and makes up an average of 20 per cent of your bodyweight. It's needed to form new tissue as well as body enzymes and hormones.

What does it do?
Protein is broken down for fuel during exercise, so you need a concentrated source of it to supplement your usual intake. Protein supplements should ideally also contain high levels of essential amino acids, which are readily digested, absorbed and retained by the body for muscle repair.

Who should take it?
All athletes need to compensate for increased breakdown of protein during training. Strength athletes need extra to provide the stimulus for muscle growth.

How much should I take?
The Food Standards Authority recommends a daily intake of 55g of protein for adults, but most dieticians agree that this isn't enough for anyone who is training regularly. The International Olympic Committee recommends around 1.2-1.4g of protein per kilo of bodyweight a day for endurance athletes or 1.4-1.7g per kilo for power athletes.

Here are the basics
If you're lean – have less than ten per cent body fat – then try to have a post-workout shake with 0.6g of protein and 1.2g of carbs per kilo of lean body weight (LBM). So an 80kg man would need roughly 43.2g of protein and 98.4g of carbs.

If you're above ten per cent body fat then the formula is the same as above, but with the amino acids L-glycine and L-glutamine in place of the carbs.

That said, if you are a serious athlete then you can't really get too much protein. Some report big benefits when eating

'Overeating protein will not make you fat and it won't hurt you unless you have kidney disease'

upwards of 3g per kilogram each day, and you won't get fat because any excess your body doesn't need gets flushed out when you pee. The only exception to this is if you have a pre-existing kidney disease. If you don't, then eat up in the knowledge that your hard work in the gym is getting the required nutritional support.

When should I take it?
The most important thing is to make sure you get some protein early in the post-exercise recovery phase, ideally immediately after exercise when your muscles need it most.

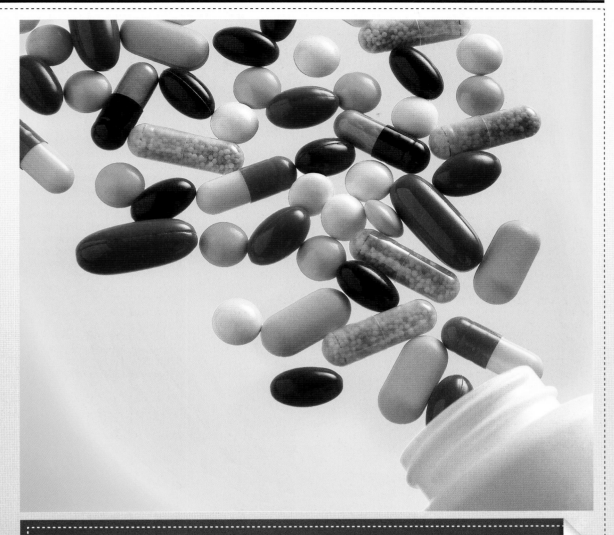

PROTEIN 101 What's going into your shake

CASEIN
Casein, which makes up 80 per cent of the protein content of milk, is made up of larger protein molecules, which are digested more slowly than whey, providing a slow, steady release of amino acids into the bloodstream. This slow release is what many experts argue makes it the best protein to use before going to sleep at night or for breakfast.

WHEY
Whey, which is derived from milk, is digested and absorbed relatively quickly, making it useful for post-exercise recovery. It also has a higher concentration of essential amino acids than whole milk, which may help minimise muscle protein breakdown immediately after exercise.

WHICH IS BEST AFTER A WORKOUT?
Why not have both? What many people forget is that you can mix your whey with casein (milk) and get both. After a workout, if you mix a 25g scoop of protein powder into a 250ml serving of milk then you've got a big chunk of fast-acting whey right when you need it, with the all the added benefits of 16g of long-acting casein.

SUPPLEMENTS

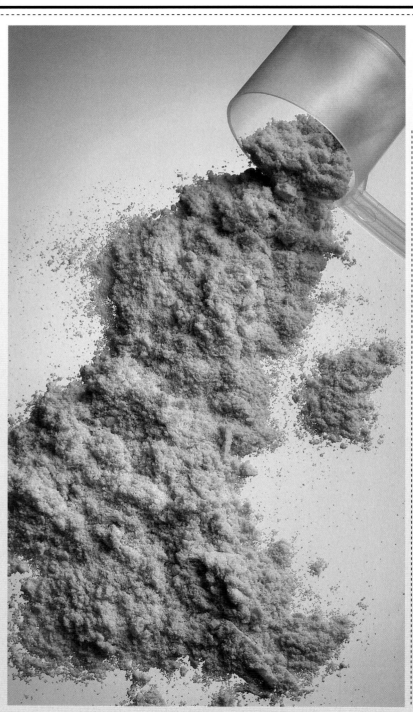

Any side effects?
It used to be thought that excess protein could place excess stress on the liver or kidneys, but this has never been demonstrated on healthy people, only those already suffering from kidney failure. A high protein intake can potentially cause dehydration – so make sure you're drinking plenty of water – but other than that it won't do you any harm.

CREATINE

What is it?
Creatine is a compound that is made naturally in the body, but can also be found in meat and fish or taken in higher doses as a supplement. It's available on its own, but you'll also sometimes see it in meal replacement shakes and other supplements.

What does it do?
It's like a back-up generator for your body. Normally, energy in your body is produced, stored, and used via a chemical called adenosine triphosphate (ATP). But at times your body can't keep up with energy demand so it needs another source of phosphates, which is where creatine comes in. Creatine also helps promote the manufacture of protein and reduces its breakdown after exercise.

Who should take it?
People who train with weights or do sports that involve repeated high-intensity movements, such as sprints, jumps or throws, are likely to see benefits. Bodybuilders often use it, as it

increases muscle hypertrophy by drawing water into muscle cells. But there's little evidence, to show that a supplement is beneficial to endurance athletes.

How much should I take?
The average man takes in 1g of creatine a day from food and produces another 1g from amino acids, resulting in creatine stores that are about 40 per cent below his maximum capacity. The best way to fill up is with doses of around 3g a day. Any more than 5g and you'll just excrete it.

When should I take it?
Avoid drinking creatine before a workout as it's hygroscopic, which basically means it acts like a sponge, drawing water into your gastrointestinal tract and bloodstream from surrounding tissues or muscles. That's what can give you a bloated feeling or sometimes muscle cramps. The ideal time to take creatine is immediately after your workout.

Any side effects?
The main side effect is weight gain. This is partly the result of increased muscle tissue but also partly because of the extra water in your muscle cells, so it's not always ideal to use it if you're competing in a sport that uses weight categories, such as boxing. There are also some, admittedly, anecdotal reports of gastrointestinal discomfort, dehydration, muscle injury and kidney damage, but there is no clinical evidence to support these statements.

GLOSSARY
Don't let yourself be dazzled by the fancy words on the label. Here's what they really mean

ANABOLISM
'Anabolic' processes build up organs and tissues, using smaller molecules to create larger ones. Anabolic steroids, for instance, increase protein synthesis in cells – although you'll see a lot of supplements that promise similar results without the side effects.

CATABOLISM
This is basically the breaking down of large molecules into smaller ones to produce energy. Products such as glutamine and antioxidants are said to reduce the rate of catabolism, meaning that you'll recover from exercise faster.

HYDROPHILIC
Substances labelled hydrophilic dissolve easily in water or blood. Normal creatine, for instance, is lipophilic, although you need to dilute it a lot.

LIPOPHILIC
Lipophilic substances pass through cell membranes easily, meaning they're absorbed quickly. Some expensive brands of creatine are more lipophilic than plain

monohydrate, which they claim makes them more effective.

LOADING
Some lifters refer to a 'loading' phase of supplement use, in which they'll take large amounts of them to build up stores in their body. This isn't always possible, however – if you take too much creatine or protein at once, for instance, your body just excretes it. Stick with the dose on the packet.

ION EXCHANGE
This basically means your protein has been separated via electrical charge, which is slightly cheaper than microfiltration. It means you'll lose some amino acids, but it also filters out a lot of fat and lactose.

MICRO FILTRATION
'Cross flow microfiltered' protein uses a very fine membrane to filtre proteins, leaving helpful amino acids intact, filtering out fat and leaving immune-boosting components untouched. On the downside, this tends to be a bit more expensive than ion-exchange-filtered protein.

AMINO ACIDS

What are they?
BCAA (branched-chain amino acids) supplements contain valine, leucine and isoleucine. These are 'essential' amino acids because they need to be present in your diet – as opposed to 'non-essential' amino acids, which your body can produce itself. Together, they can comprise up to one-third of muscle protein.

What do they do?
The theory is that they can help prevent the breakdown of muscle tissue during intense exercise. They also act to increase the release of human growth hormone.

Who should take them?
Anyone who weight trains, but opt for capsule form rather than tablet or liquid. There's little evidence that BCAAs

WHAT SUPP?

Your supplement queries answered

Can't my diet fulfil all my nutritional needs?

Yes, if you really watch what you eat. But sometimes you'll find that getting the optimum amount of certain substances for your training means eating a lot. Getting all the creatine many trainers recommend would mean eating a mountain of beef. Use supplements to fill the gaps in your diet, but don't rely on them to counteract bad eating habits.

Do I need to take supplements on the days I'm not training?

Short answer: yes. You get stronger as you recover from exercise, so making sure you're getting enough nutrients on your rest days is essential.

Should I be waking up in the middle of the night to take supplements?

Almost definitely not. You might have heard about bodybuilders getting up at 3am to neck a quick shake, but as soon as you're awake for more than three seconds you disrupt the production of melatonin, which is one of the most important hormones in building muscle. You're better off having some nice slow-digesting protein, such as raw nuts, cottage cheese or a casein shake, before bed.

Are they safe?

Since sports supplements are technically classified as food, they aren't subject to the same strict manufacturing, safety testing or labelling as licensed medicines so there's no guarantee that they'll live up to their claims. The EU is considering the introduction of stricter guidelines but it's currently up to individual manufacturers to maintain the quality of their products. Look for supplements that are ISO17025 certified, which means they've been subjected to rigorous checks during their production.

Can I fail a drugs test from taking supplements?

If you're a serious enough sportsman to be tested, then you need to be careful. A survey from an International Olympic Committee-accredited laboratory in Cologne looked for steroids in 634 supplements and found that 15 per cent of them contained substances that would cause a failed drug test, although none contained steroids. If you're concerned, consult a registered nutritionist or dietician before taking supplements.

If I take the right combination of things, can I get ripped without working out?

Sadly, no. Anyone who tells you that a magic formula can give you massive biceps and sculpted abs is fibbing. Eat right, train hard, and choose well-researched and tested supplement products, and you'll see the results you want.

will improve performance for endurance athletes, and unless you're training seriously hard you can probably get enough BCAAs from a recovery drink.

How much should I take?

The science suggests that anything less than 20 capsules per workout is a waste of time. Many professional rugby and football clubs have seen huge improvements in performance using about 40 caps of BCAAs every workout.

When should I take them?

They work best if taken before, during and post-workout. Studies have shown that taking BCAA supplements taken before resistance training reduce delayed onset muscle soreness, while taking them during and after exercise can reduce muscle breakdown.

Any side effects?

BCAAs are fairly safe, since you'd normally find them in protein in your diet anyway. Too much might reduce the absorption of other amino acids.

ANTIOXIDANTS

What are they?

Antioxidant supplements contain differing amounts of nutrients and plant extracts, including betacarotene, vitamins C and E, zinc, copper and magnesium. As well as having a beneficial effect on your general health, antioxidants can also help you recover from sports training.

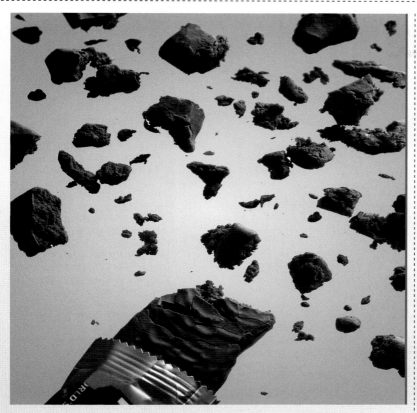

'Antioxidant supplements can protect against age-related diseases and cancer'

When should I take them?
This depends on the supplement you're taking and the effect you're looking for. Vitamin C is the antioxidant best taken after a workout because it blocks cortisol, the stress hormone. A 2008 study suggested that antioxidants are most beneficial when taken with meals – rats fed red wine alongside meat ended up with fewer free radicals in their digestive tracts than their non-drinking siblings – but the evidence isn't conclusive.

Any side effects?
There are side effects related to excessive consumption of certain vitamins found in antioxidant supplements – massive amounts of carotene can turn your skin temporarily orange, for example. Also, the antioxidant minerals zinc, magnesium and copper – can be toxic in large doses. If you stick to the recommended dosage, though, you'll be fine.

FAT BURNERS

What are they?
Also known as thermogenics, these are blends of herbs and stimulants that slightly increase your body temperature, which can help you burn more calories during exercise. Ephedrine, a synthetic version of the Chinese herb ephedra, used to be a key ingredient in these, but it's now

What do they do?
Very intense exercise can increase your body's generation of molecules known as free radicals, which can harm cell membranes, disrupt DNA and increase your risk of age-related diseases and cancer. Some evidence suggests that antioxidant supplements will protect against these diseases, though other studies suggest supplements are less effective than getting antioxidants as part of your diet. And there's not much evidence they'll actually help your sports performance.

Who should take them?
The jury is out but it has been suggested that, because of the environment and average stress levels, everyone should be on some type of antioxidant. They work best if rotated, so alternate between green tea for ten days before switching to grapeseed extract, for example.

How much should I take?
The EU recommended daily amount for vitamin C is 60mg and 10mg for vitamin E, but some scientists believe these levels are too low. Crucially, however, it's important to remember that supplements are no substitute for proper nutrition so aim to eat at least five portions of fruit and vegetables daily. Including as many different coloured fruits and vegetables as possible ensures you get the widest variety of antioxidants.

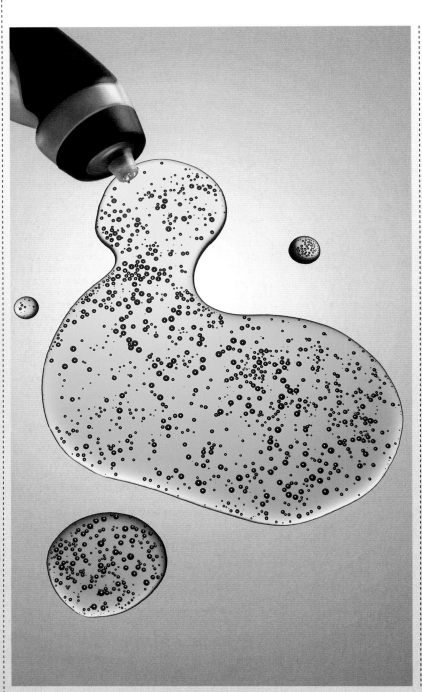

only available on prescription in the UK due to its harmful side effects and addictive qualities.

What do they do?

Some simply burn calories as heat. Others also claim to stimulate the release of adrenaline, increase your metabolic rate or act as appetite suppressants. The evidence for them working is limited, however, and a high-protein diet with regular exercise is likely to produce better weight-loss results in the long term.

Who should take them?

Fat burners raise cortisol – a stress hormone that in some cases may acutely increase abdominal fat, especially if you're already leading a fairly stressful life. In extreme cases they can cause the adrenal system to get wiped out. If you think you need them consult your GP first.

How much should I take?

Follow the instructions on the bottle, but be careful with long-term use.

When should I take them?

Most contain caffeine and so will probably make you jittery, which means that the morning's probably best time for these supplements. Never take fat burners after 2pm because they affect sleep patterns, and always follow instructions on the bottle.

Any side effects?

Taking very high doses of ephedrine can have serious effects, including palpitations, anxiety, insomnia, vomiting and dizziness. While herbal alternatives are generally safer, you may get side effects with high doses – some can raise blood pressure or even cause heart disturbances.

THE BEST OF THE REST

What else is on the shelf of your local health food shop?

CLA

Conjugated linoleic acid is an unsaturated fatty acid normally found in full-fat milk, meat and cheese. It's usually marketed as a fat-loss supplement that works by releasing fat from fat cells or blocking new fat from getting in. Experts believe it's better at the latter and recent evidence suggests that CLA works mostly by inhibiting fat-cell filling, meaning it prevents fat cells from getting larger, which is not the same as causing loss of existing body fat. CLA may therefore turn out to be more useful for preventing fat gain than for causing loss of fat you already have. Most researchers recommend 2g-5g a day, divided into three doses.

ENERGY GELS

These come in small squeezable sachets and are designed to provide an easy way of consuming carbohydrates during intense endurance exercise lasting longer than an hour. Studies have shown that they delay fatigue and increase endurance, but they aren't designed to do away with the need to carry water – you'll still need to drink around 350ml with every 25g of gel or you'll be at increased risk of dehydration.

HMB

Beta-hydroxy beta-methylbutyrate (HMB) is made in the body from BCAAs and is thought to be involved in cellular repair. Studies suggest that it may increase strength and muscle mass and reduce muscle damage after resistance exercise, although this hasn't been found in all studies. You can also find it in grapefruit.

GLUTAMINE

Glutamine is a non-essential amino acid that the body synthesises. It is needed for cell growth and as fuel for the immune system. During periods of heavy training or stress, levels of it in the body fall. There's clinical evidence that glutamine supplements can decrease your risk of infection during these periods, but less evidence that it'll actually improve your performance.

MRPS

Meal replacement products are designed to provide a good-quality meal without the hassle of cooking. A good one will contain 30-40g of protein, some good carbohydrate sources such as maltodextrin, and vitamins and minerals. It's still better to eat fresh food if you've got the time, though.

NITRIC OXIDE

The active ingredient in this is L-arginine, a non-essential amino acid made in the body. Nitric oxide is a gas involved in increasing blood flow to the muscles, delivering more nutrients and oxygen to them and theoretically causing a better pump, muscle growth and recovery. But, clinical trials haven't yet managed to prove that these supplements work.

TAURINE

This is a non-essential amino acid produced naturally in the body. You'll recognise it from Red Bull cans, but it's also found in meat, fish, eggs and milk, as well as many creatine and protein products. These regularly claim that it'll give you extra energy, but that's debatable. One review surveyed nine years of research on the National Library of Medicine's database and concluded that the energy-enhancing effects of most generic energy drinks were mainly down to the caffeine. They concluded that the 'lesser known ingredients of energy drinks — including taurine — needed further study.'

TESTOSTERONE BOOSTERS

These aim to increase testosterone levels in the body, producing similar muscle-building effects to anabolic steroids without the side effects. There's plenty of anecdotal evidence to suggest that they work, but very little in the way of proven clinical trials.

ZMA

Zinc monomethionine aspartate combines zinc, magnesium, vitamin B6 and aspartate in a formula that claims to boost testosterone. If you're training really intensely you might benefit from the extra zinc and magnesium, but don't exceed maximum doses, especially if you're using other supplements.

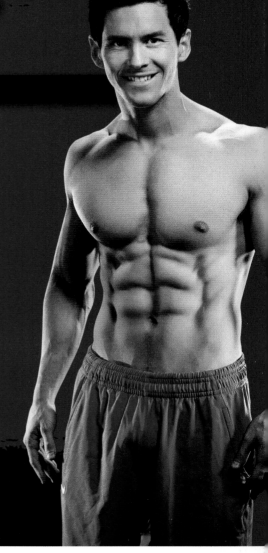

TRY 3 ISSUES FOR JUST £1

and get the body you've always wanted!

Inside *Men's Fitness*

- ➲ New workouts to help you build muscle
- ➲ Meal plans that strip away fat
- ➲ Fitness advice from leading experts
- ➲ Winning tips from top sportsmen
- ➲ Gear for active men tested and rated

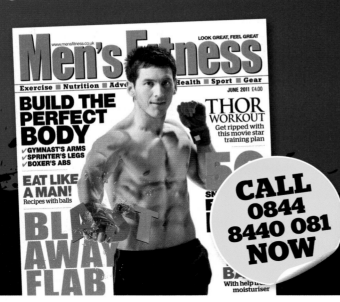

CALL 0844 8440 081 NOW

Claim 3 issues of *Men's Fitness* for £1!

Order online today at

www.dennismags.co.uk/mensfitness or

CALL 0844 844 0081

using offer code G1110RM

If during **your 3 issues**, you decide *Men's Fitness* isn't for you, simply cancel and you won't pay a penny more. But if you continue reading you'll **SAVE 16%** on the shop price, and pay just £19.95 every 6 issues.